UNLOCKING

THE

TRAUMA

TRAP

DEDICATION

To all those who have endured the pain and suffering of childhood trauma, this book is for you. Your strength and resilience in the face of unimaginable adversity inspire me every day. This book is dedicated to your courage, your tenacity, and your unyielding spirit.

May the pages of this book provide you with the tools and knowledge you need to break free from the trauma trap and reclaim your power. May it serve as a beacon of hope and a roadmap to healing.

I dedicate this book to all the survivors out there who have refused to be defined by their past, who have chosen to confront their demons head-on, and who have taken the bold and daring step on the path to a fulfilling future. This book is for you, with all my heart and soul.

TABLE OF CONTENTS

CHAPTER ONE

CHAPTER TWO

CHAPTER THREE

CHAPTER FOUR

CHAPTER FIVE

FORWARD

"Dear reader,

I am thrilled to introduce you to this transformative and empowering book, 'Unlocking the Trauma Trap: Breaking Free from the Chains of Childhood Trauma'. In these pages, you will embark on a journey of healing, growth, and liberation from the grip of childhood trauma.

Childhood trauma can be one of the most devastating experiences a person can endure, and its effects can linger long into adulthood, impacting every aspect of our lives. But the good news is that it doesn't have to be that way. With the right tools, support, and guidance, we can overcome the trauma and find our way to a brighter future.

In this book, you will discover a wealth of knowledge and insight into the nature of childhood trauma and its impact on our lives. You will learn about the different types of trauma, their root causes, and how they affect our physical, emotional, and mental health.

But more importantly, you will find practical strategies, techniques, and exercises that will help you break free from the chains of trauma and live the life you deserve. You will discover how to build resilience, cultivate self-compassion, and develop a positive mindset that will empower you to overcome adversity and thrive.

This book is not just a collection of theories and research; it is a heartfelt and compassionate guide that speaks directly to your soul. It is a roadmap to freedom, a beacon of hope, and a testament to the power of human resilience.

So, whether you are a survivor of childhood trauma, a therapist, or someone who wants to understand and support those who have suffered, this book is for you. I invite you to dive into these pages with an open heart and mind and discover the path to healing, growth, and liberation.

Sincerely,

David B. Calvin

CHAPTER ONE

CHILDHOOD TRAUMA (Introduction)

Before you begin on this journey, here are a few accounts of champions who have looked trauma in the face and said "trauma no matter how strong you think you are, you failed to see how strong and resilient i am. You only scratched the tip of the iceberg"

The Story of Jane a CHAMPION

Jane had a difficult childhood. She grew up in an abusive household where her parents were constantly fighting and shouting. Her father was an alcoholic and would often come home late at night and yell at her and her mother. Jane's mother, on the other hand, was emotionally distant and would rarely show her any affection.

As a result of this environment, Jane developed anxiety and depression at a young age. She struggled to form meaningful relationships with others and found it difficult to trust people.

However, despite the challenges she faced, Jane was determined to turn her life around. She started seeing a therapist and worked on developing coping strategies for her anxiety. She also joined a support group for survivors of childhood trauma, which helped her feel less alone and gave her a sense of community.

Over time, Jane began to make progress. She started to feel more confident in herself and was able to form meaningful relationships with others. She pursued her passion for writing and started a blog about her experiences, which helped her connect with others who were going through similar struggles.

Eventually, Jane was able to confront her past and find closure. She forgave her parents for the pain they had caused her and learned to let go of the anger and resentment she had been holding onto for so long.

Today, Jane is a successful writer and advocate for survivors of childhood trauma. She uses her platform to raise awareness about the importance of mental health and the impact of childhood trauma on adult lives. She is proof that with resilience and determination, anyone can overcome the effects of childhood trauma and live a fulfilling life.

The story of Mark a WARRIOR

As a child, Mark experienced severe physical and emotional abuse at the hands of his parents. He was constantly told that he was worthless and that he would never amount to anything. Mark grew up feeling unloved and unwanted, and this led him to develop depression and anxiety.

Despite the challenges he faced, Mark was determined to break the cycle of abuse in his family. He reached out to a counselor and started attending therapy sessions. Through therapy, Mark was able to confront the trauma he had experienced and start to heal from his past.

Mark also found solace in his passion for music. He started playing the guitar and writing songs as a way to express his emotions. Music became an outlet for Mark to release his pain and connect with others who had similar experiences.

As Mark continued to heal, he began to realize that he had a gift for helping others. He started volunteering at a local shelter for abused children, where he used his musical talents to inspire and uplift the children who were going through similar struggles as he once did.

Over time, Mark became a mentor and role model for these children. He showed them that it was possible to overcome the effects of childhood trauma and to find happiness and success in life. Mark went on to pursue a career as a counselor and worked with other survivors of childhood trauma, helping them find hope and healing in their own lives.

Today, Mark is a successful counselor and musician. He continues to inspire others with his story of resilience and serves as a reminder that anyone can overcome the effects of childhood trauma with the right support and mindset.

The story of Samantha a CONQUEROR

Samantha grew up in a household where her father was an alcoholic and her mother struggled with addiction. She was in the center of domestic violence and was exposed to substance abuse from a young age. Samantha's childhood was filled with fear and uncertainty, and as a result, she developed depression and anxiety.

Despite the challenges she faced, Samantha was determined to break the cycle of addiction and abuse in her family. She sought help from a therapist and began to attend support groups for children of alcoholics and addicts. Through these groups, Samantha found a community of people who understood what she was going through and who could support her in her journey to recovery.

Samantha also discovered a passion for running. She started training for marathons as a way to clear her mind and cope with the stress of her past. Running became a form of therapy for Samantha, and she found that the physical challenge helped her to overcome the emotional pain she had experienced.

Over time, Samantha's mental health began to improve. She started to see the world in a more positive light and felt more confident in herself. Samantha went on to pursue a career in counseling and became a mentor for other survivors of childhood trauma.

Today, Samantha is a successful counselor and marathon runner. She uses her platform to raise awareness about the impact of addiction and childhood trauma on mental health and to encourage others to seek help and support in their own journeys of recovery. Samantha's story is a testament to the resilience of the human spirit and serves as an inspiration to others who are struggling to overcome the effects of childhood trauma.

There are many more success stories of Survivors, victors and champions who have weathered the storm of childhood trauma and came out with smiles on the other side. This is just to encourage those who are going through the same or have suffered from trauma in the past that if **JANE, MARK, SAMANTHA** and a whole lot of others can do it, then why not you, mostly with the tools in this book

What is childhood trauma?

Childhood trauma is a broad term that refers to any adverse experience a child may experience, that causes physical or psychological harm, and interferes with their overall well-being. The effects of childhood trauma can be long-lasting and devastating, as it can negatively impact various aspects of an individual's life, including their mental and physical health, relationships, and overall quality of life.

Research indicates that childhood trauma is more common than one may think, and its effects can be severe and long-lasting. We will see more on the definition of childhood trauma, the types of childhood trauma, the prevalence of childhood trauma, the effects of childhood trauma, and treatment options for individuals who have experienced childhood trauma.

Definition of Childhood Trauma:

Childhood trauma refers to any experience that a child finds overwhelming or threatening to their physical, emotional, or psychological well-being. These experiences can take many forms, including abuse, neglect, witnessing violence or addiction in the home, natural disasters, and chronic illness. Childhood trauma can have long-lasting effects on a person's mental and physical health, relationships, and ability to function in society.

Types of Childhood Trauma:

There are several types of childhood trauma, including physical, sexual, and emotional abuse, neglect, and witnessing or experiencing violence. Physical abuse is when a child is physically harmed or injured by a caregiver, such as hitting, punching, or burning. Sexual abuse is when a child is exposed to any sexual activity or contact, including touching, fondling, or penetration. Emotional abuse is when a child is subjected to verbal or emotional abuse, such as humiliation, belittling, or threats. Neglect is when a caregiver fails to provide adequate care for a child's physical or emotional needs, such as food, shelter, or medical attention. Witnessing or experiencing violence can occur when a child is exposed to domestic violence, community violence, or any other violent act.

Here are some types of childhood trauma in a listed format:

- **Physical abuse:** Physical abuse refers to any form of physical harm or injury inflicted on a child by a caregiver or parent. Physical abuse can include slapping, hitting, burning, kicking, or any form of physical punishment.
- **Sexual abuse:** Sexual abuse involves any form of sexual activity that a child is forced to participate in or observe. This includes sexual contact, molestation, exploitation, exposure to pornography, or any other sexual activity that is not age-appropriate.
- **Emotional abuse:** Emotional abuse is any form of psychological harm inflicted on a child. This can include verbal abuse, belittlement, isolation, rejection, or any other form of emotional or psychological mistreatment.
- **Neglect:** Neglect refers to the failure of a caregiver to provide adequate care for a child. This can include failure to provide adequate food, clothing, shelter, medical care, supervision, or emotional support.

- **Witnessing violence:** Witnessing or being exposed to violence in the home or community can be traumatic for a child. This can include witnessing domestic violence, community violence, or any other form of violence.

- **Separation or abandonment:** Separation or abandonment can occur when a parent or caregiver is absent or unavailable for an extended period. This can include divorce, incarceration, or any other situation where a child is separated from a caregiver.

- **Medical trauma:** Medical trauma can occur when a child undergoes medical procedures or treatment that is painful or frightening. This can include surgery, hospitalization, or any other medical procedure that is traumatic for the child.

- **Natural disasters**: Natural disasters such as hurricanes, earthquakes, or floods can be traumatic for children. The loss of home, school, or community can be traumatic for a child, as well as the fear and uncertainty that can come with such events.

- **Terrorism or war:** Exposure to terrorism or war can be traumatic for children. This can include exposure to violence, death, or destruction, as well as the fear and uncertainty that can come with such events.

- **Cultural or systemic trauma:** Cultural or systemic trauma can occur when a child experiences discrimination, racism, or other forms of systemic oppression. This can include exposure to poverty, homelessness, or any other form of systemic disadvantage.

It is important to note that childhood trauma can occur in many different forms and can have a lasting impact on a child's life. If you or someone you know is experiencing childhood trauma, it is important to seek help and support from a qualified mental health professional.

Prevalence of Childhood Trauma:

Research indicates that one in four children experience some form of childhood trauma. Additionally, children who experience one form of childhood trauma are likely to experience other forms of trauma, as there is a high degree of overlap among the different types of childhood trauma.

Effects of Childhood Trauma:

The effects of childhood trauma can be devastating and long-lasting. Childhood trauma can negatively impact various aspects of an individual's life, including their mental and physical health, relationships, and overall quality of life. Some of the effects of childhood trauma include:

1. **Mental Health Issues:** Childhood trauma can increase the risk of developing mental health issues, such as depression, anxiety, post-traumatic stress disorder (PTSD), and substance abuse.

2. **Physical Health Issues:** Childhood trauma can increase the risk of developing physical health issues, such as obesity, heart disease, and chronic pain.

3. **Behavioral Issues:** Childhood trauma can lead to behavioral issues, such as aggression, impulsivity, and self-harm.

4. **Interpersonal Relationship Issues:** Childhood trauma can impact an individual's ability to form healthy relationships with others, leading to difficulties in socializing, maintaining friendships, and forming intimate relationships.

5. **Cognitive Issues:** Childhood trauma can impact an individual's cognitive development, leading to difficulties in learning, memory, and attention.

6. **Economic Issues:** Childhood trauma can negatively impact an individual's economic status, as it can

interfere with their ability to complete education or maintain employment.

It is important to note that not all children who experience trauma will have long-lasting effects, and some children are more resilient than others. However, if you or someone you know has experienced childhood trauma and is struggling with its effects, seeking professional help can be beneficial. Therapy and support groups can provide tools and strategies to cope with the trauma and move towards healing.

Childhood Trauma Impact

The impact of childhood trauma can be profound and long-lasting, affecting multiple areas of a person's life, including physical and mental health, relationships, and social functioning. In this article, we will discuss the various ways childhood trauma can affect an individual and the available interventions to mitigate these effects.

- **Physical health effects:**

Childhood trauma can have significant physical health effects, including changes in brain development and function, increased risk of chronic diseases, and alterations in the body's stress response system. Exposure to prolonged stress during childhood can cause the brain to develop differently, resulting in reduced brain volume in key areas related to learning, memory, and emotional regulation. This can contribute to difficulties with attention, memory, impulse control, and decision-making later in life. Additionally, chronic stress can impair the body's immune system, leading to an increased risk of infections and illnesses.

Childhood trauma is also associated with an increased risk of chronic diseases, including heart disease, diabetes, and obesity. The Adverse Childhood Experiences (ACE) study, a large-scale study of childhood trauma, found that individuals who had experienced four or more types of childhood trauma were at a significantly higher risk of developing these chronic diseases later in life. This may be due to the impact of stress on the body's systems, including the cardiovascular, endocrine, and immune systems.

Importantly, childhood trauma can alter the body's stress response system, leading to a heightened sensitivity to stressors later in life. This can cause individuals to experience more intense physical reactions to stress, including increased heart rate, blood pressure, and cortisol levels. Over time, this can contribute to a range of physical health problems, including cardiovascular disease, obesity, and diabetes.

- **Mental health effects**

  Childhood trauma can have significant mental health effects, including increased risk of mental health disorders, impaired social functioning, and decreased academic achievement. Traumatic experiences during childhood can lead to long-lasting changes in brain structure and function, resulting in a higher risk of developing mental health disorders, such as depression, anxiety, post-traumatic stress disorder (PTSD), and substance use disorders.

Childhood trauma can also impair social functioning, making it difficult for individuals to form and maintain healthy relationships. This can result in feelings of isolation, loneliness, and difficulty trusting others. In addition, childhood trauma can impact academic achievement, with individuals who have experienced trauma more likely to struggle with academic performance and drop out of school.

- **Relationships and social functioning**

Childhood trauma can also have significant effects on relationships and social functioning. Individuals who have experienced trauma may struggle with intimacy, trust, and communication, leading to difficulties in forming and maintaining healthy relationships. Trauma can also lead to difficulties with self-esteem and self-worth, making it challenging for individuals to develop healthy social connections. In addition, childhood trauma can impact social functioning, leading to difficulties in social situations and a higher risk of social isolation. This can contribute to feelings of loneliness, depression, and anxiety, further exacerbating the negative effects of childhood trauma.

How childhood trauma impacts adulthood

Childhood trauma can have significant and long-lasting effects on an individual's mental, physical, and emotional health, which can extend into adulthood. Here are some ways in which childhood trauma can impact adulthood:

- **Mental Health:** Childhood trauma can increase the risk of developing mental health disorders such as depression, anxiety, and post-traumatic stress disorder

(PTSD). It can also lead to the development of maladaptive coping strategies such as substance abuse, self-harm, and disordered eating.

- **Physical Health:** Childhood trauma has been linked to a higher risk of developing physical health problems such as cardiovascular disease, chronic pain, and autoimmune disorders.
- **Relationships:** Childhood trauma can make it difficult for individuals to form and maintain healthy relationships in adulthood. Trauma can cause individuals to have trust issues, difficulty with intimacy, and problems with communication.
- **Self-esteem:** Childhood trauma can negatively impact an individual's self-esteem and self-worth. Trauma can cause individuals to feel shame, guilt, and self-blame.
- **Career:** Childhood trauma can impact an individual's career by making it difficult for them to maintain employment or advance in their careers. Trauma can cause individuals to struggle with concentration, motivation, and decision-making.

It is important to seek professional help if you have experienced childhood trauma and are experiencing negative impacts on your mental, physical, and emotional health in adulthood. Therapy, support groups, and other forms of treatment can be effective in helping individuals heal from childhood trauma and improve their overall well-being. The effects shall be extensively discussed in the following chapter.

CHAPTER TWO

ACE STUDY SUMMARY

Adverse childhood experiences (ACE) study:

This study was conducted by the Centers for Disease Control and Prevention (CDC) and Kaiser Permanente between 1995 and 1997. The study focused on identifying and understanding the impact of childhood adversity on adult health outcomes.

The ACE study identified some of the following types of childhood trauma that are considered adverse childhood experiences. These experiences includes:

- **Physical abuse**

- **Emotional abuse**

- **sexual abuse**

- **emotional neglect**

- **parental divorce or separation**

- **a parent with a mental illness**

- **Substance use disorder**

- **Witnessing domestic violence.**

The study found that the more ACEs an individual had experienced, the higher the likelihood of developing health problems later in life.

The study found that over 60% of the 17,000 participants reported experiencing at least one ACE, and over 20% reported experiencing three or more ACEs. The study also found that individuals who experienced four or more ACEs were more likely to experience negative health outcomes, including chronic diseases such as heart disease, diabetes, and cancer. They were also more likely to engage in risky behaviors such as smoking, substance abuse, and unprotected sex.

The ACE study highlights the importance of understanding the impact of childhood trauma on adult health outcomes. The study suggests that childhood trauma is a significant public health concern and should be addressed with appropriate interventions. The study also emphasizes the need for healthcare providers to be aware of the impact of childhood trauma on their patients' health and to ask about childhood experiences during routine health screenings.

In conclusion, the Adverse Childhood Experiences study has shed light on the relationship between childhood trauma and adult health outcomes. The study's findings have important implications for public health and emphasize the need for early intervention and prevention strategies to mitigate the negative impact of childhood trauma.

How to prevent childhood trauma from ever occurring

Childhood trauma is a serious issue that affects millions of children worldwide. Trauma can result from many different sources, including abuse, neglect, violence, and natural disasters. The effects of childhood trauma can be long-lasting and can affect a child's physical, emotional, and mental health.

Preventing childhood trauma from ever occurring is crucial to ensure that children can grow up healthy and resilient. Here are some strategies that parents, caregivers, and communities can implement to prevent childhood trauma:

- **Build strong and positive relationships**: Strong and positive relationships are crucial for a child's healthy development. Parents, caregivers, and other adults in a child's life should strive to build positive relationships with children that are based on trust, respect, and empathy. Positive relationships can help children develop a sense of security and stability, which can protect them from trauma.

- **Provide a safe and stable environment:** Children need a safe and stable environment to thrive. Parents and caregivers should ensure that children have access to safe housing, food, and clothing. They should also provide a stable home environment by setting clear boundaries, providing routine and structure, and modeling healthy behaviors.

- **Address mental health issues:** Mental health issues such as depression and anxiety can increase the risk of childhood trauma. Parents and caregivers should be aware of the signs and symptoms of mental health issues and seek professional help when necessary. Early intervention can help prevent mental health issues from escalating and leading to trauma.

- **Address substance abuse:** Substance abuse is a major risk factor for childhood trauma. Parents and caregivers should avoid using drugs and alcohol in the presence of children and seek professional help if they have a substance abuse problem. Children who grow up in households with substance abuse are at a higher risk of experiencing trauma.

- **Provide education and support:** Education and support can help parents and caregivers prevent childhood trauma. Parents and caregivers should be educated on the signs and symptoms of trauma and how to prevent it. They should also be provided with resources and support to help them cope with stress and parenting challenges.

- **Promote resilience:** Parents and caregivers can help children develop resilience by providing them with opportunities to develop coping skills, problem-solving skills, and emotional regulation skills. Children who are resilient are better able to cope with stress and adversity, which can protect them from trauma.

- **Address societal factors:** Many societal factors, such as poverty, racism, and inequality, can increase the risk of childhood trauma. Communities can work to address these factors by advocating for policies that promote social justice and equality. Parents and caregivers can also work to address these factors by advocating for their children's rights and providing them with opportunities to learn about and engage in social justice issues.

It is important to understand that preventing childhood trauma from ever occurring is crucial for ensuring that children can grow up healthy and resilient. Parents, caregivers, and communities can implement strategies such as building strong and positive relationships, providing a safe and stable environment, addressing mental health issues, addressing substance abuse, providing education and support, fostering resilience, and addressing societal factors to prevent childhood trauma. By working together, we can create a world where children can thrive and reach their full potential.

Common causes of childhood trauma

Childhood trauma is a complex and multifaceted phenomenon that can have profound and lasting effects on a child's emotional, psychological, and physical well-being. Childhood trauma refers to any event, circumstance, or experience that poses a significant threat to a child's physical or emotional safety or well-being. Traumatic experiences can range from physical, sexual, and emotional abuse, to neglect, exposure to violence, or the death of a loved one.

While every child's experience is unique, there are some common causes of childhood trauma that are worth exploring in greater detail.

1. **Abuse:** Abuse is one of the most common causes of childhood trauma. Physical abuse involves the use of physical force or violence, such as hitting, slapping, or shaking a child. Sexual abuse involves any sexual act between an adult and a child, including sexual contact, penetration, or exposure to sexual images or materials. Emotional abuse, on the other hand, refers to any behavior or treatment that causes emotional harm to a child, such as verbal abuse, intimidation, or constant criticism.

2. **Neglect:** Neglect is another common cause of childhood trauma. It occurs when a child's basic needs for food, shelter, clothing, medical care, or supervision are not met. Neglect can take many forms, including physical neglect (e.g., inadequate food, shelter, or medical care), emotional neglect (e.g., lack of affection or attention), and educational neglect (e.g., failure to provide adequate schooling or support).

3. **Exposure to violence:** Children who are exposed to violence are at risk of developing traumatic stress reactions. This can include witnessing violence in the home, community, or media, as well as experiencing violence directly. Exposure to violence can include

physical abuse, sexual abuse, bullying, or witnessing violent behavior in others.

4. **Family conflict:** Family conflict can also be a source of childhood trauma. This can include parents who fight or argue frequently, divorce or separation, or conflict between siblings. Family conflict can be particularly traumatic for children, as they may feel caught in the middle or powerless to change the situation.

5. **Medical trauma:** Children who experience medical trauma, such as a serious illness, hospitalization, or invasive medical procedures, may also be at risk of developing traumatic stress reactions. Medical trauma can be particularly traumatic for children, as they may experience significant pain, discomfort, or anxiety during these procedures.

6. **Natural disasters:** Natural disasters, such as hurricanes, earthquakes, and floods, can also be a source of childhood trauma. These events can be particularly traumatic for children, as they may feel powerless or out of control during the event and may have difficulty understanding or coping with the aftermath.

7. **Accidents and injuries:** Accidents and injuries can also be a source of childhood trauma. This can include

car accidents, falls, or other types of accidents that result in injury or harm. Children who experience accidents or injuries may be at risk of developing traumatic stress reactions, especially if the event was particularly violent or traumatic.

8. **Loss of a loved one:** The loss of a loved one, whether it be a parent, grandparent, sibling, or pet, can be a significant source of childhood trauma. Children may struggle to understand or cope with the loss, and may experience feelings of grief, sadness, and anxiety.

9. **Migration and displacement:** Children who are forced to migrate or flee their homes due to war, persecution, or other forms of violence may also be at risk of experiencing childhood trauma. These children may experience significant stress and anxiety during the migration process, as well as in the new environment they find themselves in.

10. **Systemic oppression and discrimination:** Children who experience systemic oppression and discrimination, such as racism or sexism, are very likely to develop trauma both physically and mentally.

Childhood Trauma Symptoms:

Childhood trauma is a distressing experience that occurs before the age of 18 and has a significant impact on a person's mental, physical, and emotional health. Childhood trauma can result from many different experiences, including physical, sexual, or emotional abuse, neglect, witnessing violence, natural disasters, and family conflicts.

The signs and symptoms of childhood trauma can vary widely and may depend on the type, frequency, and severity of the trauma, as well as the child's age, gender, and individual temperament. In this article, we will explore the most common signs and symptoms of childhood trauma, how they may manifest in different age groups, and the long-term effects of childhood trauma.

Emotional symptoms

Emotional symptoms are some of the most common signs of childhood trauma. Some of the following symptoms can be found in children who have experienced trauma:

- **Anxiety and fear:** Children who have experienced trauma may become overly anxious and fearful about specific situations, people, or objects. They may experience panic attacks, have difficulty sleeping, or develop phobias.

- **Depression:** Children who have experienced trauma may become depressed and have feelings of hopelessness, worthlessness, and sadness. They may also have a lack of interest in activities they previously enjoyed and may withdraw from social interactions.

- **Anger and irritability:** Children who have experienced trauma may be easily angered and irritable. They may lash out at others, be defiant or disobedient, and have difficulty controlling their emotions.

- **Shame and guilt:** Children who have experienced trauma may experience feelings of shame and guilt, even if they are not responsible for the trauma. They may feel as if they are flawed, unlovable, or unworthy of happiness.

Behavioral symptoms

Behavioral symptoms are another common indicator of childhood trauma. Children who have experienced trauma may exhibit the following behavioral symptoms:

- **Regression:** Children who have experienced trauma may regress to earlier stages of development. For example, a child who has been potty-trained may start wetting the bed again or start sucking their thumb.

- **Avoidance:** Avoidance refers to a child's efforts to avoid anything that might trigger memories or reminders of the traumatic event. Children who have experienced trauma may exhibit avoidance by avoiding certain people, places, or activities, or by engaging in avoidance behaviors such as substance abuse, overeating, or isolating themselves from others.

- **Hypervigilance:** Hypervigilance refers to a state of heightened awareness and sensitivity to potential danger. Children who have experienced trauma may exhibit hypervigilance by being overly cautious or fearful in everyday situations, or constantly scanning their environment for potential threats.

- **Self-destructive behaviors:** Children who have experienced trauma may engage in self-destructive behaviors, such as substance abuse, self-harm, or risky sexual behavior.

Cognitive symptoms

Cognitive symptoms refer to the way a child thinks and processes information. Children who have experienced trauma may exhibit the following cognitive symptoms:

- **Poor memory:** Children who have experienced trauma may have difficulty remembering things, especially if the trauma occurred at a young age.

- **Difficulty with attention and concentration:** Children who have experienced trauma may have trouble paying attention or staying focused on tasks.

- **Negative self-image:** Children who have experienced trauma may have a negative self-image and believe that they are responsible for the trauma or that they are inherently flawed.

- **Distorted beliefs about the world:** Children who have experienced trauma may develop negative beliefs about the world and the people in it. For example, they may believe that the world is a dangerous place, or that they cannot trust anyone.

Physical symptoms

Physical symptoms are another possible indicator of childhood trauma. Children who have experienced trauma may exhibit the following physical symptoms:

- **Headaches and stomachaches:** Children who have experienced trauma may complain of frequent headaches or stomach aches, even when there is no underlying medical condition.
- **Sleep disturbances:** Children who have experienced trauma may have difficulty falling asleep or staying asleep. They may also experience nightmares.
- **Chronic pain:** Children who have experienced trauma may experience chronic pain, such as headaches, stomachaches, or muscle pain.
- **Poor health:** Children who have experienced trauma may have more frequent illnesses or experience a decline in their overall health.

Social symptoms

Social symptoms refer to a child's ability to interact with others and form relationships. Children who have experienced trauma may exhibit the following social symptoms:

- **Difficulty forming attachments:** Children who have experienced trauma may have difficulty forming attachments to caregivers or other adults. They may also have difficulty trusting others.

- **Isolation:** Children who have experienced trauma may isolate themselves from others and avoid social situations.

- **Poor social skills:** Children who have experienced trauma may have difficulty with social skills, such as sharing, taking turns, or communicating their needs.

- **Aggression towards others:** Children who have experienced trauma may display aggression towards others, such as hitting, biting, or pushing.

Sexual symptoms

Sexual symptoms may be present in children who have experienced sexual abuse or assault. These symptoms may include:

- **Inappropriate sexual behaviors:** Children who have experienced sexual trauma may engage in inappropriate sexual behaviors, such as touching themselves or others inappropriately, or mimicking sexual acts.

- **Sexualized play:** Children who have experienced sexual trauma may engage in sexualized play or make sexual comments that are not appropriate for their age.
- **Fear or avoidance of sexual activity:** Children who have experienced sexual trauma may experience fear or avoidance of sexual activity, even as they get older.

Developmental symptoms

Developmental symptoms refer to the child's ability to reach developmental milestones. Children who have experienced trauma may exhibit the following developmental symptoms:

- **Delayed development:** Children who have experienced trauma may have delays in reaching developmental milestones, such as walking, talking, or toilet training.
- **Poor academic performance:** Children who have experienced trauma may have difficulty with academic performance and may struggle to keep up with their peers.
- **Difficulty with problem-solving:** Children who have experienced trauma may have difficulty with problem-solving and may struggle to think logically or make decisions.

Substance abuse

Substance abuse may be a symptom of childhood trauma, particularly if the trauma is related to substance abuse or if the child is using drugs or alcohol to cope with the trauma.

Eating disorders: Eating disorders, such as anorexia or bulimia, may be present in children who have experienced trauma, particularly if the trauma is related to body image or food.

It's important to note that not all children who have experienced trauma will exhibit all of these symptoms. Additionally, some children may exhibit symptoms that are not listed here. If you are concerned that a child may have experienced trauma, it's important to seek help from a mental health professional who can provide an accurate diagnosis and treatment.

Emotional dysregulation

Emotional dysregulation refers to difficulty regulating one's emotions. Children who have experienced trauma may exhibit the following emotional dysregulation symptoms:

- **Mood swings:** Children who have experienced trauma may exhibit mood swings or have rapid changes in mood.

- **Intense emotions:** Children who have experienced trauma may have intense emotional reactions, such as anger, sadness, or fear, which are difficult to manage.

- **Emotional numbing:** Children who have experienced trauma may exhibit emotional numbing, or a lack of emotion, as a way to cope with overwhelming feelings.

- **Negative self-image:** Children who have experienced trauma may have negative thoughts about themselves or believe that they are to blame for the traumatic event.

Self-harm

Self-harm refers to intentional harm to oneself. Children who have experienced trauma may engage in self-harm as a way to cope with overwhelming emotions or to feel a sense of control. Self-harm behaviors may include cutting, burning, or scratching oneself.

- **Suicidal thoughts or behaviors:** Children who have experienced trauma may experience suicidal thoughts or engage in suicidal behaviors.

- **Dissociation:** Dissociation refers to a disconnection from oneself, one's surroundings, or reality. Children who have experienced trauma may dissociate as a way to cope with overwhelming emotions or to detach from the traumatic event. Dissociation may manifest as spacing out, feeling disconnected from one's body, or feeling like one is watching oneself from outside the body.

- **Regression:** Regression refers to a child's return to earlier developmental stages or behaviors. Children who have experienced trauma may exhibit regression as a way to cope with the stress and anxiety of the trauma. For example, a child may revert to thumb-sucking, bed-wetting, or baby talk.

- **Guilt or shame:** Children who have experienced trauma may experience feelings of guilt or shame, believing that they are somehow responsible for the traumatic event or that they could have done something to prevent it. These feelings may be reinforced by negative self-trauma. For example, a child may revert to thumb-sucking, bed-wetting, or baby talk.

- **Guilt or shame:** Children who have experienced trauma may experience feelings of guilt or shame, believing that they are somehow responsible for the traumatic event or that they could have done something to prevent it. These feelings may be reinforced by negative self

CHAPTER THREE

Physical health effects of childhood trauma

From the previous chapter, a little has been mentioned on the effects of childhood trauma. In this chapter a more detailed effect of childhood trauma as it affects the various facets of life will be discussed. Childhood trauma can have a significant impact on an individual's physical health, both in childhood and throughout their life. The reason for talking about these effects in detail is to stress on the severity of Childhood Trauma and the need to tackle it.

Here are some of the physical health effects of childhood trauma:

- **Brain development:** Childhood trauma can have a significant impact on brain development. Trauma can cause changes in the structure and function of the brain, particularly in areas related to stress and emotion regulation. This can lead to long-term difficulties with impulse control, emotion regulation, and decision-making.

- **Cardiovascular health:** Childhood trauma has been linked to an increased risk of heart disease, stroke, and other cardiovascular problems. This may be due in part to the impact of trauma on stress hormones, which can lead to inflammation and other changes in the body that contribute to cardiovascular disease.

- **Immune system:** Childhood trauma can weaken the immune system, making individuals more vulnerable to infections and illnesses. This is due in part to the impact of trauma on stress hormones, which can suppress the immune system.

- **Chronic pain:** Childhood trauma has been linked to an increased risk of chronic pain in adulthood. This may be due in part to changes in the way the brain processes pain signals.

- **Substance abuse:** Childhood trauma is a significant risk factor for substance abuse in adulthood. Individuals who have experienced trauma may be more likely to use drugs or alcohol as a way to cope with the emotional and psychological effects of the trauma.

- **Sleep disturbances:** Childhood trauma can disrupt sleep patterns and lead to sleep disturbances, including nightmares and insomnia. This can contribute to a range of physical health problems, including fatigue, irritability, and difficulties with concentration and memory.

- **Obesity:** Childhood trauma has been linked to an increased risk of obesity in adulthood. This may be due in part to changes in the way the body processes food and stores fat.

- **Reproductive health**: Childhood trauma can have a significant impact on reproductive health. Trauma can disrupt the functioning of the hypothalamic-pituitary-adrenal (HPA) axis, which plays a key role in the regulation of the reproductive system. This can lead to irregular menstrual cycles, infertility, and other reproductive health problems.

- **Increased risk of chronic illnesses:** Childhood trauma has been linked to a higher risk of developing chronic illnesses, such as heart disease, diabetes, and autoimmune disorders.

- **Altered stress response:** Trauma can alter a person's stress response, making them more likely to experience chronic stress and inflammation, which can lead to a host of physical health problems.

- **Digestive problems:** Childhood trauma has been linked to digestive problems such as irritable bowel syndrome (IBS), ulcers, and other gastrointestinal disorders.

- **Hormonal imbalances:** Trauma can disrupt the balance of hormones in the body, leading to problems such as irregular menstrual cycles, infertility, and thyroid disorders.

- **Developmental delays:** In cases of severe or prolonged trauma, developmental delays can occur in children, affecting physical growth and cognitive development.

- **Self-harm:** Trauma can increase the risk of self-harm behaviors such as cutting, burning, and other forms of self-injury.

- **Sexual dysfunction:** Trauma can lead to sexual dysfunction in both men and women, including decreased libido, erectile dysfunction, and difficulty achieving orgasm.

- **Lifespan:** Childhood trauma can shorten lifespan. Studies have shown that individuals who have experienced childhood trauma have a higher risk of premature death from a range of causes, including heart disease, cancer, and suicide.

It is important to note that not all individuals who experience childhood trauma will experience these physical health effects, and the severity of the effects can vary depending on the nature and severity of the trauma, as well as individual differences.

Mental health effects of childhood trauma

Childhood trauma refers to any experience that a child perceives as emotionally or physically threatening, overwhelming, or harmful. Traumatic experiences during childhood can have a profound impact on mental health and emotional well-being, leading to a range of short- and long-term effects.

Here are some of the detailed mental health effects of childhood trauma:

- **Post-Traumatic Stress Disorder (PTSD):** Children who have experienced trauma may develop PTSD, a condition characterized by persistent, distressing thoughts and memories related to the traumatic event, as well as symptoms like nightmares and flashbacks.
- **Depression:** Childhood trauma can lead to depression, characterized by feelings of sadness, hopelessness, and a loss of interest in previously enjoyed activities. Children may also experience

changes in appetite, sleep disturbances, and difficulty concentrating.

- **Anxiety:** Childhood trauma can cause anxiety disorders. Children may experience intense fear, worry, and apprehension, along with physical symptoms such as sweating, trembling, and palpitations.
- **Attachment Issues:** Children who have experienced trauma may have difficulty forming healthy attachments to caregivers, leading to feelings of detachment, mistrust, and isolation.
- **Substance Abuse:** Children who experience trauma may be at a higher risk of developing substance abuse disorders as a way to cope with the emotional pain and distress associated with their experiences.
- **Self-Harm:** Childhood trauma can lead to self-harming behaviors such as cutting, burning, or hitting oneself as a way to cope with emotional pain and distress.
- **Eating Disorders:** Trauma can also contribute to the development of eating disorders, including anorexia, bulimia, and binge eating disorder. Children may use food as a way to cope with emotional distress or as a way to gain control over their lives.

- **Personality Disorders:** Childhood trauma can increase the risk of developing personality disorders, including borderline personality disorder and antisocial personality disorder. These conditions are characterized by difficulties with emotion regulation, impulsivity, and interpersonal relationships.

- **Dissociative Disorders:** Children who experience trauma may develop dissociative disorders, including dissociative amnesia, depersonalization disorder, and dissociative identity disorder. These conditions involve a disruption in a person's normal sense of identity, memory, or consciousness as a way to cope with overwhelming emotions or experiences.

- **Sleep Disorders:** Childhood trauma can lead to sleep disturbances, including difficulty falling or staying asleep, nightmares, and night terrors. These sleep disturbances can further contribute to mental health issues such as anxiety and depression.

- **Cognitive Impairment:** Childhood trauma can affect a child's cognitive development, leading to difficulties with attention, concentration, and memory. This can impact academic performance and overall functioning in daily life.

- **Aggression and Anger Issues:** Children who experience trauma may exhibit aggressive and impulsive behaviors, including physical and verbal outbursts, as a way to cope with their emotions and experiences

Behavioral effects of childhood trauma

Childhood trauma can have a wide range of behavioral effects, which can vary depending on the type and severity of the trauma, the age at which it occurred, and the individual's coping mechanisms. Some of the common behavioral effects of childhood trauma include:

- **Avoidance and withdrawal:** Individuals who have experienced childhood trauma may avoid situations or activities that trigger memories of the traumatic event. They may also withdraw from social situations and have difficulty forming close relationships.
- **Hyper-arousal:** Childhood trauma can lead to heightened levels of anxiety and hypervigilance. This may manifest as difficulty sleeping, irritability, and being easily startled.
- **Emotional dysregulation:** Trauma can interfere with the development of emotional regulation skills,

leading to intense and unpredictable mood swings. Individuals may struggle to identify and manage their emotions, leading to frequent outbursts or emotional shutdowns.

- **Self-destructive behaviors:** Trauma can increase the risk of engaging in self-destructive behaviors, such as substance abuse, self-harm, and reckless behavior.
- **Aggression and hostility:** Childhood trauma can lead to feelings of anger, resentment, and aggression towards others. Individuals may have difficulty controlling their impulses and may lash out in response to perceived threats or triggers.
- **Dissociation:** Trauma can lead to feelings of detachment and dissociation from reality. Individuals may have difficulty connecting with their emotions or experiences, leading to a sense of numbness or disconnection from their surroundings.
- **Difficulty with trust and attachment:** Childhood trauma can interfere with the development of trust and attachment, leading to difficulty forming close relationships or relying on others for support.
- **Negative self-image:** Trauma can lead to feelings of shame, guilt, and low self-worth. Individuals may

struggle with self-esteem and self-confidence, leading to negative self-talk and a negative self-image.

Social effects of childhood trauma

Childhood trauma can have a profound impact on an individual's social development, leading to various social effects that can persist throughout their lives. Here are some of the detailed social effects of childhood trauma:

- **Difficulty in forming and maintaining relationships:** Individuals who have experienced childhood trauma may find it challenging to form and maintain healthy relationships with others. They may have trust issues, fear of rejection or abandonment, and difficulty in expressing their emotions.

- **Emotional instability:** Childhood trauma can cause emotional instability, leading to frequent mood swings, anxiety, depression, and other mental health issues. This can negatively affect an individual's ability to interact with others and form healthy social connections.

- **Aggression and violence:** Childhood trauma can lead to aggressive and violent behavior, which can cause significant social problems. Such behavior can lead to the breakdown of relationships, physical fights, and legal issues.

- **Substance abuse:** Childhood trauma can increase the risk of substance abuse, as individuals may turn to drugs or alcohol as a coping mechanism. This can lead to addiction, which can further impair an individual's social functioning.

- **Social withdrawal:** Childhood trauma can lead to social withdrawal and isolation, as individuals may feel unsafe or unwelcome in social settings. This can further exacerbate the problem, leading to feelings of loneliness and depression.

- **Poor academic performance:** Childhood trauma can negatively affect an individual's academic performance, leading to poor grades, truancy, and dropouts. This can limit their social opportunities and future prospects.

- **Difficulty in achieving career goals:** Childhood trauma can also affect an individual's career goals and achievements. They may struggle to hold down a job or advance in their career due to emotional instability, poor social skills, or a lack of confidence.

- **Difficulty in trusting others:** Childhood trauma can lead to a lack of trust in others, which can make it challenging to form close relationships. Individuals who have experienced trauma may have a heightened sense of danger and may struggle to believe that others have their best interests at heart.

- **Negative self-image:** Childhood trauma can negatively impact an individual's self-image, leading to low self-esteem and a negative self-concept. This can affect their social interactions by making them feel inferior to others, unworthy of love or respect, and hesitant to engage with others.

- **Codependency:** Childhood trauma can lead to codependency, which is an unhealthy reliance on others to meet one's emotional needs.

- **Difficulty in managing emotions:** Childhood trauma can make it challenging to manage emotions, which can lead to outbursts or impulsive behavior. Individuals may find it challenging to regulate their emotions, leading to strained relationships with friends, family, and coworkers.

- **Trust issues with authority figures:** Childhood trauma can lead to trust issues with authority figures such as teachers, employers, or law enforcement officials. Individuals may be reluctant to follow rules, express their opinions, or seek help when needed, which can negatively impact their social and professional interactions.

- **Social anxiety:** Childhood trauma can lead to social anxiety, which is an intense fear of social situations. Individuals may feel anxious or panicked when in social situations, which can lead to avoidance behavior, social isolation, and difficulty forming relationships.

- **Difficulty with intimacy:** Childhood trauma can make it challenging for individuals to form intimate relationships. They may struggle to trust others or feel vulnerable with them, leading to difficulties with emotional and physical intimacy.

- **Self-isolation:** Childhood trauma can cause individuals to isolate themselves from others, leading to a lack of social support and increased feelings of loneliness and despair.

- **Anger and hostility:** Childhood trauma can lead to anger and hostility, making it challenging for individuals to connect with others. They may be quick to anger and respond aggressively to perceived threats, leading to social conflicts.

- **Compromised social skills:** Childhood trauma can negatively impact social skills, making it difficult for individuals to communicate effectively, empathize with others, or navigate social situations. This can lead to social difficulties in both personal and professional relationships.

- **Difficulty with boundaries:** Childhood trauma can lead to difficulty with boundaries, making it challenging for individuals to set healthy limits and maintain healthy relationships. They may struggle with asserting themselves and may allow others to take advantage of them.

- **Shame and guilt:** Childhood trauma can lead to feelings of shame and guilt, making it challenging for individuals to interact with others without feeling unworthy or inadequate. This can lead to self-imposed social isolation and difficulty forming and maintaining relationships.

- **Lack of social support:** Childhood trauma can lead to a lack of social support, as individuals may struggle to form and maintain healthy relationships. This can further exacerbate the negative effects of trauma, making it challenging for individuals to cope and heal.

In summary, childhood trauma can lead to a range of social effects, including difficulties in forming relationships, emotional instability, aggression and violence, substance abuse, social withdrawal, poor academic performance, difficulty achieving career goals, trust issues, negative self-image, codependency, difficulty managing emotions, trust issues with authority figures, and social anxiety. It's important to seek professional help if you or someone you know has experienced childhood trauma, as early intervention can help mitigate the negative effects of trauma.

CHAPTER 4

OVERCOMING CHILDHOOD TRAUMA

Childhood trauma can have a significant impact on a person's life, but it is possible to overcome its effects. Childhood trauma can take many forms, including physical, emotional, or sexual abuse, neglect, and witnessing violence or substance abuse. These experiences can lead to a variety of mental health issues, including depression, anxiety, and post-traumatic stress disorder (PTSD).

Overcoming childhood trauma is a process that requires time, effort, and support from others. Some of the following strategies can be of help:

- **Seek professional help:** Talking to a mental health professional who specializes in trauma can be a crucial step in overcoming childhood trauma. They can help you work through the emotions and memories associated with the trauma, develop coping mechanisms, and address any mental health issues that may have arisen.

- **Practice self-care:** Taking care of yourself is essential when healing from childhood trauma. Some of the self-care tips include getting adequate sleep, healthy eating, engaging in recreational activities and other activities that bring you pleasure. Connect with others: Building supportive relationships with family, friends, or a therapist can help you feel less alone and provide a source of comfort and support. Joining a support group with others who have experienced similar trauma can also be helpful.

- **Practice mindfulness:** Mindfulness practices such as meditation, yoga, or deep breathing can help you become more aware of your thoughts and emotions and learn to manage them in a healthy way.

- **Challenge negative thoughts:** Childhood trauma can leave negative beliefs about yourself and the world around you. Challenging these thoughts and replacing them with more positive ones can help you develop a more optimistic outlook.

- **Set boundaries:** Learning to say no to situations that may trigger your trauma can be an important step in protecting your emotional well-being.

- **Forgive yourself:** It is important to recognize that you are not to blame for the trauma you experienced. Forgive yourself for any perceived shortcomings or mistakes that you may have made in response to the trauma.

Overcoming childhood trauma can be a long and difficult journey, but it is possible. With time, support, and the right tools, you can heal from the effects of childhood trauma and move forward in life with confidence and resilience

Understanding childhood trauma-informed care:

Childhood trauma-informed care is a model of care that recognizes the impact of childhood trauma on individuals and seeks to provide a supportive and healing environment. Childhood trauma is any experience or event that is perceived as threatening or dangerous and that overwhelms a child's ability to cope.

Examples of childhood trauma include physical, sexual, or emotional abuse; neglect; witnessing violence or substance abuse; or experiencing a natural disaster or a serious accident.

Trauma can have long-lasting effects on a child's physical, emotional, and mental health. These effects can include depression, anxiety, post-traumatic stress disorder (PTSD), substance abuse, self-harm, and suicidal thoughts.

Childhood trauma-informed care aims to create an environment that promotes healing and recovery by addressing the effects of trauma in a compassionate and understanding way. The following are some key principles of childhood trauma-informed care:

- **Safety**: Creating a safe environment is the first step in providing trauma-informed care. The child must feel safe and secure in their environment, and they must trust their caregivers to provide them with the support they need.

- **Trustworthiness**: It is important to be honest, transparent, and consistent in all interactions with the child. This includes being reliable and following through on commitments.

- **Collaboration**: The child should be involved in the decision-making process and be given a voice in their own care. Collaboration between the child, their caregivers, and other professionals involved in their care is key.

- **Empowerment**: Providing the child with the tools and resources they need to feel empowered and in control of their own healing process is important. This can include giving them a sense of autonomy and choice in their care.

- **Cultural sensitivity:** It is important to understand and respect the child's cultural background and to incorporate cultural beliefs and practices into their care.

- **Strengths-based:** Focusing on the child's strengths rather than their deficits is important in promoting healing and recovery. This includes recognizing and building on the child's resilience and coping skills.

- **Trauma-informed practices:** Trauma-informed practices include recognizing the signs and symptoms of trauma, understanding the impact of trauma on development, and providing interventions that are evidence-based and trauma-sensitive.

- **Understanding the impact of trauma:** Trauma can affect individuals in many different ways, and it is important to understand the impact of trauma on development and functioning. Trauma can affect a child's ability to regulate emotions, form relationships, and engage in academic and social activities.

- **Providing trauma-specific interventions:** Trauma-specific interventions are evidence-based treatments that are designed to address the specific symptoms and effects of trauma. These interventions include cognitive-behavioral therapy, trauma-focused cognitive-behavioral therapy, and eye movement desensitization and reprocessing (EMDR).

- **Addressing the effects of trauma in schools:** Childhood trauma can affect a child's ability to learn and succeed in school. Trauma-informed schools provide a safe and supportive environment for students and recognize the impact of trauma on learning and behavior.

- **Building resilience:** Resilience is the ability to recover from adversity and to adapt to new situations. Building resilience is an important part of childhood trauma-informed care and involves promoting the child's strengths and coping skills.

- **Providing support to caregivers:** Caregivers play a critical role in supporting children who have experienced trauma. Providing support to caregivers can include education about trauma and its effects, assistance with accessing services and resources, and support for self-care.

- **Fostering a trauma-informed culture:** Fostering a trauma-informed culture involves creating a culture of safety, support, and understanding. This can involve training and education for staff and professionals, as well as creating policies and procedures that support trauma-informed care.

Implementing childhood trauma-informed care requires a multidisciplinary approach that involves caregivers, mental health professionals, educators, and other professionals. It is important to provide training and education to all individuals involved in the care of children to ensure that they understand the principles of trauma-informed care and how to implement them in their practice.

In summary, childhood trauma-informed care is a model of care that recognizes the impact of childhood trauma on individuals and seeks to provide a supportive and healing environment. It involves creating a safe, trustworthy, collaborative, empowering, culturally sensitive, strengths-based, and trauma-informed environment. By implementing these principles, individuals who have experienced childhood trauma can begin to heal and recover in a supportive and compassionate environment.

Professional help for childhood trauma victims

Childhood trauma can have long-lasting effects on a person's mental health and well-being. Seeking professional help is an important step in the healing process for childhood trauma victims. In this article, we will explore the benefits of seeking professional help, the different types of therapy available, and what to expect during the therapy process.

Benefits of Seeking Professional Help

Childhood trauma can manifest in a variety of ways, including depression, anxiety, PTSD, and substance abuse. Seeking professional help can help childhood trauma victims address these issues and develop coping mechanisms to manage their symptoms.

Professional help can also provide a safe space for childhood trauma victims to explore their emotions and experiences without judgment. This can be particularly important for victims who may have been told to keep their experiences a secret or who feel shame about what has happened to them.

Different Types of Therapy Available

There are several different types of therapy that childhood trauma victims can benefit from. Some common types of therapy include:

- **Cognitive-behavioral therapy (CBT)**

- **Eye Movement Desensitization and Reprocessing (EMDR)**
- **Play therapy**
- **Art therapy, etc.**

What to Expect During the Therapy Process

The therapy process can vary depending on the type of therapy and the individual's specific needs. However, there are some general things that childhood trauma victims can expect during the therapy process:

- **Assessment:** The therapist will likely conduct an initial assessment to gather information about the individual's experiences and symptoms.
- **Goal-setting:** The therapist and individual will work together to set goals for the therapy process.
- **Treatment:** The therapist will use different techniques and strategies to help the individual process their experiences and develop coping mechanisms.
- **Follow-up:** The therapist may follow up with the individual to monitor progress and make adjustments to the treatment plan if necessary.

The professional help for overcoming childhood trauma shall be discussed in detail in the next chapter.

Self-help strategies for victims of childhood trauma

Experiencing childhood trauma can have a profound impact on a person's mental and emotional well-being, but there are self-help strategies that can help victims of childhood trauma cope and heal. Here are some suggestions:

1. **Seek support:** Talk to someone you trust about your experiences, such as a friend, family member, or therapist. Having a support system can help you feel less alone and provide you with a safe space to process your emotions.

2. **Educate yourself:** Learn more about childhood trauma and how it affects people. Understanding the ways that trauma can impact your life can help you better cope with its effects.

3. **Set boundaries:** It is important to establish boundaries to protect yourself from further harm. This could mean limiting contact with people who trigger

negative emotions or situations that bring up difficult memories.

4. **Express yourself creatively:** Art therapy, writing, or other creative outlets can help you express your emotions in a safe and healthy way.

5. **Practice mindfulness:** Mindfulness techniques, such as deep breathing or meditation, can help you stay present in the moment and reduce anxiety.

6. **Consider seeking professional help:** A therapist or counselor can help you work through your trauma and develop coping strategies to manage its effects.

7. **Practice self-compassion:** Be kind and gentle with yourself. Treat yourself with the same love and understanding that you would offer to a close friend. Recognize that healing from trauma is a process and it takes time.

8. **Develop a self-soothing toolkit:** Identify activities or things that comfort and calm you, such as listening to music, taking a warm bath, or cuddling with a pet. Have a list of these activities on hand for when you are feeling overwhelmed.

9. **Connect with others who have experienced similar trauma:** Joining a support group or finding a community of people who have experienced similar

trauma can help you feel less alone and provide you with a sense of understanding and belonging.

10. **Practice grounding techniques:** Grounding techniques can help you feel more present and connected to the present moment. For example, focusing on your breathing, noticing five things you can see, four things you can touch, three things you can hear, two things you can smell, and one thing you can taste.

11. **Create a safety plan:** Develop a plan for what to do if you feel triggered or unsafe. This could include identifying safe places to go, people to contact, and coping strategies to use.

12. **Practice forgiveness:** Forgiving those who have harmed you can be a difficult process, but it can also be a powerful tool for healing. Remember that forgiveness is not about excusing harmful behavior, but about letting go of the anger and resentment that can hold you back.

13. **Engage in advocacy or activism:** Taking action to promote awareness of childhood trauma or working to prevent it from happening to others can be empowering and healing.

14. **Practice gratitude:** Cultivating gratitude can help you shift your focus away from negative thoughts and emotions. Take time each day to reflect on things you are grateful for, no matter how small.

15. **Build a positive identity:** Childhood trauma can lead to feelings of shame and low self-worth. Working on building a positive sense of self can help counteract these negative beliefs. This could include focusing on your strengths, setting goals, and practicing self-compassion.

16. **Learn relaxation techniques:** Relaxation techniques, such as progressive muscle relaxation or guided imagery, can help reduce anxiety and promote relaxation.

17. **Practice assertiveness:** Childhood trauma can make it difficult to set boundaries and speak up for yourself. Practicing assertiveness can help you develop these skills and feel more empowered.

18. **Engage in physical activity**: Find an activity that you enjoy, whether it's running, yoga, or dancing just ensure that you don't stay idle.

19. **Practice self-reflection:** Take time to reflect on your experiences and emotions. Journaling or talking to a

trusted friend or therapist can help you process your thoughts and feelings.

Remember that these strategies are not a substitute for professional help. If you are struggling with the effects of childhood trauma, consider reaching out to a therapist or counselor for additional support.

Remember that healing from childhood trauma is a journey, and it's important to be patient with yourself. These strategies can be helpful, but if you are struggling with the effects of trauma, seeking professional help is always a good option.

Building a support system for overcoming childhood trauma

Overcoming childhood trauma can be a long and difficult journey, but building a strong support system can make a significant difference. Here are some steps you can take to build a support system:

1. **Seek professional help:** A trained therapist or counselor can provide you with the guidance, tools, and support you need to overcome your childhood trauma. They can help you develop coping strategies, identify triggers, and work through painful emotions.

2. **Join a support group:** Joining a support group can be a great way to connect with others who have experienced similar trauma. Being able to share your experiences with others who understand what you're going through can be incredibly healing.

3. **Build a network of supportive friends and family:** Surround yourself with people who support and encourage you. Friends and family can provide emotional support, help you stay motivated, and provide a sense of belonging.

4. **Practice self-care:** This could include things like eating well, getting enough sleep, exercising regularly, and practicing mindfulness or meditation.

5. **Find creative outlets:** Engage in activities that bring you joy, such as painting, writing, or playing music.

Remember, building a support system takes time and effort. With the right support, you can heal from your childhood trauma and live a happy, fulfilling life

Types of therapy for victims of childhood trauma

There are several types of therapy that can be helpful for individuals who have experienced childhood trauma. Here are some examples:

Cognitive Behavioral Therapy (CBT): CBT focuses on identifying and changing negative thought patterns and behaviors that may be contributing to mental health problems related to trauma. It can also involve exposure therapy, where the individual is gradually exposed to the source of their trauma in a safe and controlled environment to help them overcome their fears.

Eye Movement Desensitization and Reprocessing (EMDR): EMDR is a type of therapy that focuses on reprocessing traumatic memories using bilateral stimulation, such as eye movements, sounds, or touch. The goal is to help the individual process the traumatic memory in a way that reduces its impact on their mental health.

Dialectical Behavior Therapy (DBT): DBT is a type of therapy that helps individuals develop coping skills to manage intense emotions and improve relationships. It can be helpful for individuals who have experienced trauma and struggle with emotional regulation.

Trauma-focused Cognitive Behavioral Therapy (TF-CBT): It focuses on helping individuals process their trauma and develop coping skills to manage symptoms related to trauma.

Mindfulness-based Therapies: These types of therapies, such as mindfulness-based stress reduction (MBSR) and mindfulness-based cognitive therapy (MBCT), can help individuals develop awareness and acceptance of their thoughts and emotions related to trauma. It can also help individuals develop coping skills to manage stress and anxiety related to trauma.

It's important to note that different types of therapy may be more or less effective for different individuals, and it may take some trial and error to find the right type of therapy or combination of therapies that work for each person. It's also important to seek out a qualified therapist who has experience working with individuals who have experienced trauma.

Psychodynamic Therapy: This type of therapy focuses on exploring unconscious thoughts and past experiences to help individuals gain insight into their emotions, behaviors, and relationships. It can be helpful for individuals who have experienced trauma and may be struggling with unresolved emotional conflicts.

Narrative Therapy: Narrative therapy involves exploring the stories individuals tell themselves about their experiences and identities. This type of therapy can help individuals reframe their experiences of trauma and develop a more positive and empowering narrative.

Art Therapy: Art therapy involves using art to express emotions and explore feelings related to trauma. It can be helpful for individuals who have difficulty expressing themselves verbally or who may be hesitant to talk about their trauma.

Yoga Therapy: Yoga therapy involves using yoga postures, breathing techniques, and mindfulness practices to help individuals manage symptoms related to trauma. It can be helpful for individuals who have experienced trauma and may be struggling with anxiety or depression.

Group Therapy: Group therapy involves working with a therapist and other individuals who have experienced trauma in a supportive and safe environment. It can help individuals feel less isolated and provide opportunities to connect with others who may have similar experiences. Group therapy can also be a cost-effective option for individuals who may not be able to afford individual therapy.

It's important to remember that every individual's experience of trauma is unique, and what works for one person may not work for another. It's important to work with a qualified therapist to develop a personalized treatment plan that takes into account an individual's specific needs and goals.

The various types of therapies shall be discussed in detail in the following chapter.

CHAPTER FIVE

THERAPIES FOR CHILDHOOD TRAUMA

In this part we shall see in detail some of the therapies available for victims of childhood trauma, the components of the therapy and what to expect in the course of the therapy. It is also important to note that therapies are highly effective, because they can awaken self-consciousness and stir up within the ability to heal thus overcoming the effects of childhood trauma.

COGNITIVE BEHAVIORAL THERAPY FOR CHILDHOOD TRAUMA

Cognitive-behavioral therapy (CBT) is a type of talk therapy that has been shown to be effective in treating childhood trauma. CBT for childhood trauma focuses on helping the child or adolescent identify and change negative thoughts, beliefs, and behaviors that may be perpetuating their trauma-related symptoms.

CBT for childhood trauma typically consists of several components, including:

1. **Psychoeducation:** The therapist will educate the child and their family about trauma and its effects on the brain and body.

2. **Cognitive Restructuring:** This involves identifying and changing negative or distorted thoughts and beliefs that may be causing distress. The therapist may use techniques such as cognitive restructuring or thought records to help the child challenge their negative thoughts and beliefs.

3. **Exposure Therapy:** This involves gradually exposing the child to trauma-related stimuli in a safe and controlled environment, allowing them to process and eventually overcome their fear or anxiety related to the trauma.

4. **Relaxation Techniques:** These techniques can help the child manage stress and anxiety related to the trauma. Examples may include deep breathing, progressive muscle relaxation, or mindfulness.

5. **Behavioral Activation:** This involves encouraging the child to engage in positive activities and behaviors that can help them feel better and improve their mood. CBT has been shown to be effective in reducing trauma-related symptoms in children and adolescents. Studies have found that CBT can improve mood, reduce

anxiety and depression, and improve relationships with family and peers.

Tailoring CBT to the Child's Needs

CBT for childhood trauma is tailored to meet the individual needs of each child. The therapist will work closely with the child and their family to identify specific goals for therapy and develop a treatment plan that addresses their unique needs.

Building Trust and Safety

Building a trusting and safe therapeutic relationship is essential in CBT for childhood trauma. The therapist will work to establish a sense of safety and trust with the child, which can help them feel comfortable sharing their experiences and emotions.

Family Involvement

Family involvement is an important aspect of CBT for childhood trauma. The therapist will work with the child's family to help them understand and support the child's treatment goals. Family members may be involved in therapy sessions or may be provided with education and support outside of therapy.

Integration with Other Treatment Approaches

CBT for childhood trauma may be used in combination with other treatment approaches, such as medication or other therapies. The therapist may work with the child's healthcare provider to ensure that treatment is coordinated and effective.

Effectiveness of CBT for Childhood Trauma

Research has shown that CBT is an effective treatment for childhood trauma. A meta-analysis of 12 randomized controlled trials found that CBT was effective in reducing symptoms of PTSD, anxiety, and depression in children and adolescents who had experienced trauma.

Limitations of CBT for Childhood Trauma

CBT may not be effective for all children or may require more than one approach to fully address the child's needs. Some children may also require longer-term therapy or additional support to fully recover from their trauma.

CBT is a highly effective treatment for childhood trauma that can help children and adolescents overcome negative thoughts and beliefs related to their trauma. By tailoring treatment to meet the child's individual needs, building a safe and trusting therapeutic relationship, involving the child's family, and integrating other treatment approaches as needed, CBT can help children and adolescents recover from their trauma and lead healthy, happy lives.

While cognitive-behavioral therapy (CBT) has been shown to be effective in treating childhood trauma, there are some limitations to this approach. Here are some of the limitations of CBT for childhood trauma:

Limited Focus on Emotions

CBT primarily focuses on cognitive and behavioral changes, but may not address the emotional aspects of trauma as comprehensively as other therapies. This may limit the effectiveness of CBT for children who have experienced severe or complex trauma, as they may need additional support to process and cope with their emotions.

Limited Exploration of Trauma History

CBT may not provide enough time or space for the child to explore their trauma history in depth. This may limit the effectiveness of CBT for children who have experienced complex trauma or have multiple traumas, as they may need more time and support to process and integrate their experiences.

Requires Active Participation

CBT requires the child to actively participate in therapy and engage in homework assignments outside of sessions. This may be challenging for some children, especially those who are resistant to therapy or have limited support at home.

Limited Cultural Sensitivity

CBT may not fully address cultural differences in beliefs, values, and attitudes toward trauma and mental health. This may limit the effectiveness of CBT for children from diverse cultural backgrounds, who may benefit from more culturally sensitive approaches.

Limited Access to Skilled Therapists

CBT requires skilled therapists with specialized training in trauma and CBT techniques. However, many children and families may not have access to such therapists, especially in rural or low-income areas.

May Not Address Comorbid Conditions

CBT may not effectively address comorbid conditions, such as substance abuse or personality disorders, which may be common among individuals who have experienced childhood trauma. These conditions may require additional treatment or support to effectively manage.

In conclusion, while CBT is an effective treatment approach for childhood trauma, it may have limitations in addressing emotions, exploring trauma history, requiring active participation, addressing cultural differences, limited access to skilled therapists, and not addressing comorbid conditions. Other therapeutic approaches, such as play therapy, expressive arts therapy, or trauma-focused therapy, may be necessary to fully address the needs of children who have experienced childhood trauma.

EMDR THERAPY FOR CHILDHOOD TRAUMA

(Eye movement desensitization and reprocessing therapy on childhood trauma)

Eye Movement Desensitization and Reprocessing (EMDR) therapy is a psychotherapeutic intervention that has been shown to be effective in treating a variety of mental health conditions, including post-traumatic stress disorder (PTSD), anxiety, and depression. EMDR therapy involves a series of structured sessions in which the therapist guides the client through a process of reprocessing traumatic memories while simultaneously engaging in eye movements or other forms of bilateral stimulation. In this write-up, we will explore the application of EMDR therapy specifically to childhood trauma.

Childhood trauma is a significant public health issue that affects millions of people worldwide. Trauma experienced during childhood can have lasting effects on mental health and well-being, and can impact a person's ability to form healthy relationships, regulate their emotions, and function effectively in day-to-day life. EMDR therapy has been shown to be an effective treatment for childhood trauma, particularly when it is delivered in a structured and supportive environment by a trained professional.

The EMDR therapy process typically involves eight phases, although the number of sessions and the specific details of the treatment may vary depending on the individual needs of the client.

The first phase of EMDR therapy involves an initial assessment, during which the therapist and client work together to identify specific traumatic memories or experiences that are causing distress. This assessment may involve the use of standardized questionnaires or other assessment tools to help the therapist gain a better understanding of the client's history and current symptoms.

The second phase of EMDR therapy involves preparation and stabilization. This phase is designed to help the client develop coping strategies and emotional regulation skills to help manage any distress or discomfort that may arise during the treatment process. The therapist may teach the client relaxation techniques, mindfulness exercises, and other self-soothing techniques to help them manage any anxiety or other difficult emotions that may arise.

The third phase of EMDR therapy involves the actual reprocessing of traumatic memories. During this phase, the therapist guides the client through a series of eye movements or other forms of bilateral stimulation while asking them to focus on the traumatic memory or experience. This process is designed to help the client desensitize to the traumatic memory and reprocess it in a way that reduces its emotional impact and helps the client gain a more adaptive perspective on the experience.

The fourth through seventh phases of EMDR therapy involve further reprocessing of traumatic memories and the integration of new insights and perspectives. The therapist may ask the client to focus on related memories or experiences and engage in additional bilateral stimulation to help desensitize and reprocess these memories. The therapist may also help the client identify new beliefs or perspectives that are more adaptive and helpful, and work with the client to integrate these new beliefs into their daily life.

The final phase of EMDR therapy involves closure and evaluation. During this phase, the therapist and client review the progress that has been made during the treatment process and identify any remaining issues or concerns that may need to be addressed. The therapist may also help the client develop a plan for managing any future triggers or difficulties that may arise.

Research has shown that EMDR therapy is effective in treating childhood trauma. A systematic review and meta-analysis of randomized controlled trials of EMDR therapy for children and adolescents with PTSD found that EMDR therapy was more effective than control conditions and at least as effective as other active treatments such as cognitive-behavioral therapy (CBT) and play therapy. A study by de Roos and colleagues (2011) found that EMDR therapy was effective in reducing symptoms of PTSD, depression, and anxiety in children who had experienced sexual abuse. Another study by Ironson and colleagues (2002) found that EMDR therapy was effective in reducing symptoms of PTSD and depression in children who had experienced Hurricane Andrew.

A study by Chemtob and colleagues (2000) found that EMDR therapy was effective in reducing symptoms of PTSD in children who had experienced a variety of traumatic events, including physical abuse, sexual abuse, and witnessing violence. The study found that the effects of EMDR therapy were maintained at a 6-month follow-up assessment.

Another study by Diehle and colleagues (2015) examined the effectiveness of EMDR therapy in treating children who had experienced multiple traumas. The study found that EMDR therapy was effective in reducing symptoms of PTSD, depression, and anxiety, and that these effects were maintained at a 6-month follow-up assessment.

A systematic review and meta-analysis of studies on EMDR therapy for children and adolescents with PTSD found that EMDR therapy was effective in reducing symptoms of PTSD, depression, and anxiety, and that these effects were maintained at follow-up assessments (Bae et al., 2018). The review also found that EMDR therapy was effective in improving overall functioning and quality of life.

EMDR therapy has been found to be particularly effective in treating childhood trauma because it addresses the underlying neural and physiological mechanisms that are involved in trauma. Traumatic experiences are stored in the brain in a disorganized and fragmented manner, making it difficult for the individual to integrate the experience into their overall understanding of themselves and the world. EMDR therapy works to reorganize and integrate these memories, allowing the individual to process the trauma in a more adaptive way.

Additionally, EMDR therapy has been found to be effective in reducing the symptoms of dissociation, which is a common response to childhood trauma. Dissociation is a coping mechanism in which the individual mentally separates themselves from their experiences, often resulting in a feeling of detachment or numbness. EMDR therapy helps the individual to reconnect with their experiences in a safe and controlled way, allowing them to process the trauma and integrate it into their overall understanding of themselves and the world.

Overall, EMDR therapy is a promising intervention for childhood trauma that has been found to be effective in reducing symptoms of PTSD, depression, and anxiety, and improving overall functioning and quality of life. It is important to note, however, that EMDR therapy is not appropriate for everyone and should only be delivered by a trained professional. It is important to work with a qualified therapist to determine the most appropriate treatment approach for your specific needs and circumstances.

Summarized list of the benefits of EMDR

- **Effective in reducing symptoms of PTSD, depression, and anxiety:** EMDR therapy has been found to be effective in reducing symptoms of PTSD, depression, and anxiety in individuals who have experienced trauma.
- **Improves overall functioning and quality of life:** EMDR therapy has been found to improve overall functioning and quality of life in individuals who have experienced trauma.

- **Addresses underlying neural and physiological mechanisms of trauma:** EMDR therapy works to reorganize and integrate traumatic memories, allowing the individual to process the trauma in a more adaptive way.

- **Reduces symptoms of dissociation:** EMDR therapy helps individuals to reconnect with their experiences in a safe and controlled way, allowing them to process the trauma and integrate it into their overall understanding of themselves and the world.

- **Can be a relatively short-term intervention:** EMDR therapy is often a relatively short-term intervention compared to other forms of therapy, with some individuals experiencing significant improvement in symptoms in just a few sessions.

- **Can be used in combination with other therapies:** EMDR therapy can be used in combination with other therapies, such as cognitive-behavioral therapy, to address the complex needs of individuals who have experienced trauma.

Limitations of EMDR therapy

While EMDR therapy has been found to be an effective intervention for childhood trauma, it is important to consider its limitations as well. Some potential limitations of EMDR therapy include:

- **Lack of research on long-term outcomes:** While several studies have found that EMDR therapy is effective in reducing symptoms of PTSD and other psychological disorders in the short-term, there is limited research on the long-term outcomes of EMDR therapy. It is important to consider the potential for relapse or the need for ongoing therapy after completing EMDR treatment.

- **Potential for re-traumatization:** EMDR therapy involves revisiting traumatic memories, which can be emotionally challenging and potentially re-traumatizing for some individuals. A trained therapist can help to manage these potential risks by providing support and guidance throughout the treatment process.

- **Limited access to trained therapists:** EMDR therapy requires specialized training and certification, which can limit access to qualified therapists in some areas. This can make it difficult for individuals to access this treatment approach.

- **Not suitable for all individuals**: EMDR therapy may not be suitable for all individuals, particularly those with certain medical or psychological conditions. It is important to work with a qualified therapist to determine if EMDR therapy is appropriate for your specific needs and circumstances.

- **Potential side effects:** Some individuals may experience side effects from EMDR therapy, such as headaches, dizziness, or anxiety. These side effects are usually mild and short-lived, but it is important to discuss any concerns with your therapist.

In summary, while EMDR therapy has been found to be an effective intervention for childhood trauma, it is important to consider its potential limitations and risks. Working with a qualified therapist and discussing any concerns can help to ensure that EMDR therapy is a safe and effective treatment approach for your specific needs and circumstances.

It is important to work with a qualified therapist to determine the most appropriate treatment approach for your specific needs and to discuss any potential risks or limitations of EMDR therapy.

DBT FOR CHILDHOOD TRAUMA

(Dialectical behavior therapy on childhood trauma)

DBT is an evidence-based therapy that focuses on teaching individuals skills to manage difficult emotions, improve interpersonal relationships, and tolerate stressful situations. Dialectical behavior therapy consists of the following modules:

1. Mindfulness

The mindfulness module in DBT teaches individuals to be present in the moment and observe their thoughts, emotions, and bodily sensations without judgment. Mindfulness helps individuals to develop awareness of their internal experiences, which can help them regulate their emotions and reduce stress. Mindfulness exercises such as deep breathing, body scans, and meditation are often used in DBT.

2. Distress Tolerance

The distress tolerance module in DBT teaches individuals how to tolerate and manage stressful situations without engaging in self-destructive behaviors such as self-harm or substance use.

Distraction involves redirecting attention away from the distressing situation by engaging in activities such as exercise, listening to music, or reading. Self-soothing involves using sensory stimuli such as sight, sound, touch, taste, or smell to provide comfort and relaxation. Radical acceptance involves accepting reality as it is without judgment or trying to change it.

3. Emotion Regulation

The emotion regulation module in DBT teaches individuals how to identify and regulate their emotions. Emotion regulation skills include identifying emotions, reducing emotional vulnerability, and changing emotions when necessary.

Identifying emotions involves recognizing and labeling one's emotions. Reducing emotional vulnerability involves increasing positive emotions and decreasing negative emotions through activities such as self-care and practicing gratitude. Changing emotions when necessary involves using skills such as opposite action, problem-solving, and cognitive restructuring.

4. Interpersonal Effectiveness

The interpersonal effectiveness module in DBT teaches individuals how to communicate effectively and assertively, set boundaries, and maintain healthy relationships. Interpersonal effectiveness skills include assertiveness, validation, and active listening.

Assertiveness involves expressing one's needs and opinions in a clear and respectful manner. Validation involves acknowledging and validating the feelings and experiences of others. Active listening involves paying attention to and understanding what others are saying.

Application of DBT in Childhood Trauma

DBT can be an effective treatment for childhood trauma as it provides individuals with the skills to manage difficult emotions, tolerate stressful situations, and improve interpersonal relationships. DBT can be used in individual therapy, group therapy, or a combination of both.

Individual Therapy

Individual therapy involves one-on-one sessions with a therapist. In individual therapy, the therapist works with the individual to identify and address specific trauma-related issues. The therapist may use techniques such as exposure therapy, cognitive restructuring, and skill-building to help the individual manage their emotions and improve their functioning.

Exposure therapy involves gradually exposing the individual to the traumatic memory or situation in a safe and controlled environment. This can help the individual to process the trauma and reduce the intensity of their emotional response to it.

Summarized list of benefits of Dialectical Behavior Therapy (DBT) for childhood trauma:

- **Reduces emotional dysregulation:** DBT teaches skills to manage difficult emotions and regulate emotional responses, which can reduce the intensity and frequency of emotional dysregulation.
- **Improves interpersonal relationships:** DBT teaches skills to communicate effectively, set boundaries, and maintain healthy relationships, which can improve interpersonal functioning and reduce social isolation.
- **Increases distress tolerance:** DBT teaches skills to tolerate stressful situations without engaging in self-destructive behaviors, which can reduce the risk of self-harm and substance use.
- **Enhances mindfulness:** DBT teaches skills to be present in the moment and observe internal experiences without judgment, which can increase self-awareness and reduce reactivity to triggers.

- **Improves self-esteem:** DBT can help individuals to identify and challenge negative self-beliefs and develop a more positive self-concept, which can improve self-esteem and reduce self-criticism.

- **Reduces symptoms of PTSD:** DBT can be effective in reducing symptoms of post-traumatic stress disorder (PTSD) by teaching skills to manage triggers and process traumatic memories in a safe and controlled environment.

- **Provides a supportive environment:** DBT can be delivered in group therapy settings, which can provide a supportive and validating environment for individuals to share their experiences and receive peer support.

- **Promotes long-term recovery:** DBT is a skills-based therapy that teaches individuals to manage ongoing challenges and maintain recovery over the long term, which can improve overall functioning and quality of life.

TF-CBT FOR CHILDHOOD TRAUMA

(Trauma focused cognitive behavioral therapy for childhood trauma)

TF-CBT is designed to address the emotional, cognitive, and behavioral responses that can occur as a result of trauma, and it is considered to be one of the most effective treatments for childhood trauma.

Theoretical Foundations of TF-CBT

TF-CBT is based on several theoretical frameworks, including cognitive-behavioral therapy (CBT), attachment theory, and trauma theory. CBT is a widely used treatment approach that focuses on changing maladaptive thoughts and behaviors, and it has been applied to a range of mental health problems, including depression, anxiety, and posttraumatic stress disorder (PTSD).

Attachment theory posits that the relationships we form in childhood with caregivers play a critical role in our development and well-being. Trauma theory, on the other hand, suggests that exposure to traumatic events can have a profound impact on our psychological functioning, including our thoughts, emotions, and behaviors.

TF-CBT combines these theoretical perspectives to address the impact of traumatic events on children's functioning, with a particular emphasis on addressing maladaptive cognitions and behaviors that may have developed as a result of the trauma. By targeting these areas, TF-CBT aims to reduce symptoms of PTSD, depression, anxiety, and other mental health problems commonly associated with childhood trauma.

Key Principles of TF-CBT

TF-CBT is a structured, time-limited treatment approach that typically consists of 12-16 sessions. The treatment is delivered by trained mental health professionals who have expertise in working with children and adolescents.

The following are some of the key principles of TF-CBT:

- **Psychoeducation:** The first phase of TF-CBT involves providing the child and their caregiver(s) with education about trauma and its effects. This includes explaining the nature of trauma, its impact on thoughts and emotions, and how it can lead to maladaptive behaviors.
- **Relaxation skills:** Children who have experienced trauma often experience high levels of anxiety, which can make it difficult for them to engage in therapy. To address this, TF-CBT incorporates relaxation skills such

as deep breathing, progressive muscle relaxation, and guided imagery.

- **Cognitive restructuring:** TF-CBT focuses on identifying and challenging maladaptive thoughts and beliefs that may have developed as a result of the trauma. This involves teaching the child to recognize when they are engaging in negative self-talk and replacing these thoughts with more positive and realistic ones.

- **Trauma narrative:** One of the core components of TF-CBT is the trauma narrative, which involves helping the child to process their traumatic experience by telling their story in a structured and supportive environment. This process can help the child to gain a better understanding of what happened, develop a sense of mastery over the experience, and reduce the emotional intensity of the trauma.

- **Gradual exposure:** TF-CBT also incorporates gradual exposure to the traumatic event, which involves helping the child to confront the memories and emotions associated with the trauma in a safe and controlled manner. This exposure is typically done in a gradual and systematic way, starting with less distressing aspects of the trauma and building up to more challenging aspects over time.

- **Skill-building:** Finally, TF-CBT emphasizes skill-building in areas such as communication, problem-solving, and emotion regulation. These skills can help the child to cope with stressors and challenges that may arise in the future.

Techniques Used in TF-CBT

Here are some additional details about the techniques used in TF-CBT:

- **Cognitive restructuring:** This technique involves helping the child to identify and challenge negative and unrealistic thoughts that may be contributing to their emotional distress. The therapist will work with the child to replace these thoughts with more accurate and helpful ones, which can help to reduce symptoms of anxiety and depression.
- **Exposure therapy:** This technique involves gradually exposing the child to the memories and emotions associated with the traumatic event in a safe and controlled environment. This exposure can help the

child to process the trauma and reduce the intensity of their emotional reactions to it.

- **Relaxation techniques:** TF-CBT incorporates a range of relaxation techniques, such as deep breathing, progressive muscle relaxation, and guided imagery. These techniques can help the child to manage feelings of anxiety and promote a sense of calm.

- **Parenting skills training:** TF-CBT involves working with parents or caregivers to teach them skills to support their child's recovery. These skills may include techniques for promoting positive behavior, improving communication, and providing emotional support.

- **Social skills training:** This technique involves helping the child to develop skills for interacting with others in a positive and effective way. Social skills training can be particularly helpful for children who have experienced social isolation or difficulty in forming relationships as a result of their trauma.

- **Art therapy:** TF-CBT may incorporate art therapy techniques to help the child to express themselves and process their emotions in a nonverbal way. Art therapy can be particularly helpful for children who have difficulty verbalizing their feelings or who struggle with traditional talk therapy.

Research on TF-CBT

TF-CBT has been extensively researched and has been found to be effective for a range of trauma-related problems in children and adolescents. Studies have shown that TF-CBT can lead to significant reductions in symptoms of PTSD, depression, and anxiety, as well as improvements in overall functioning and quality of life.

Challenges Associated with TF-CBT

Despite its effectiveness, TF-CBT can be challenging to implement in real-world settings. One of the main challenges is identifying children who have experienced trauma and may benefit from the treatment. Many children who have experienced trauma may not seek treatment, or may be difficult to reach through traditional mental health services.

In addition, TF-CBT requires specialized training and expertise on the part of the therapist, which may not be widely available in all areas. There may also be cultural or linguistic barriers that make it difficult to deliver TF-CBT effectively to children from diverse backgrounds.

Finally, TF-CBT requires a significant time commitment on the part of both the child and their caregiver(s), which may be difficult for some families to manage. However, research suggests that the benefits of TF-CBT may outweigh these challenges, and that the treatment can lead to significant improvements in the lives of children who have experienced trauma.

TF-CBT is a highly effective treatment approach for children and adolescents who have experienced trauma. By combining cognitive-behavioral, attachment, and trauma theories, TF-CBT addresses the emotional, cognitive, and behavioral responses that can occur as a result of trauma, and helps children to develop skills for coping with these challenges. Although there are challenges associated with implementing TF-CBT, the treatment has been extensively

Summarized list of benefits of trauma focused cognitive behavioral therapy (TF-CBT):

- **Reduced symptoms of PTSD:** TF-CBT has been found to significantly reduce symptoms of post-traumatic stress disorder (PTSD) in children and adolescents who have experienced trauma.
- **Improved mood and emotional regulation:** TF-CBT can help children and adolescents to better

regulate their emotions and reduce symptoms of depression and anxiety.

- **Better functioning in daily life:** By helping children to process and cope with their trauma, TF-CBT can improve their overall functioning and quality of life.

- **Improved relationships:** TF-CBT can help children to develop better social and communication skills, which can improve their relationships with family, friends, and peers.

- **Increased sense of safety and control:** Through techniques such as exposure therapy and cognitive restructuring, TF-CBT can help children to feel more in control of their thoughts and emotions, and to develop a greater sense of safety and security.

- **Improved parenting skills:** By working with parents or caregivers, TF-CBT can help them to better support their child's recovery and develop positive parenting strategies.

- **Long-term benefits:** TF-CBT has been found to have lasting effects, with many children continuing to show improvement in symptoms and functioning even after the end of treatment.

MINDFULNESS-BASED THERAPIES FOR TRAUMA

Childhood trauma is a significant public health concern that can have long-lasting effects on an individual's mental and physical health. Mindfulness-based therapies have shown promise in helping individuals with trauma-related symptoms to manage their emotions, decrease anxiety and depression, and improve their overall well-being. This article will explore mindfulness-based therapies and their effectiveness in treating childhood trauma.

What is Mindfulness?

It is about being aware of our thoughts, feelings, and bodily sensations in the moment without getting caught up in them or reacting to them. Mindfulness can be practiced through various techniques such as breathing exercises, body scans, and mindful movement practices like yoga or Tai Chi.

Mindfulness-Based Therapies

Mindfulness-based therapies are a type of psychotherapy that incorporates mindfulness techniques into the treatment approach. These therapies are designed to help individuals develop a greater sense of awareness of their thoughts and emotions, and to learn how to manage them in a more effective way. There are several mindfulness-based therapies that have been developed to treat trauma-related symptoms, including:

- **Mindfulness-Based Stress Reduction (MBSR):** This is an eight-week program that was originally developed to help individuals with chronic pain. It has since been adapted for use with individuals experiencing trauma-related symptoms. MBSR focuses on mindfulness meditation, body awareness, and gentle yoga exercises.

- **Mindfulness-Based Cognitive Therapy (MBCT):** MBCT was developed to treat individuals with depression. It combines mindfulness techniques with cognitive-behavioral therapy (CBT) to help individuals identify and change negative thought patterns that contribute to their depression.

- **Mindfulness-Oriented Recovery Enhancement (MORE):** MORE is a newer mindfulness-based therapy that was developed to treat individuals with addiction. It combines mindfulness techniques with positive psychology and cognitive-behavioral therapy to help individuals develop a greater sense of meaning and purpose in their lives.

Effectiveness of Mindfulness-Based Therapies for Childhood Trauma

A 2017 meta-analysis of 12 studies on the effectiveness of mindfulness-based interventions for trauma-related symptoms found that these therapies were effective in reducing symptoms of post-traumatic stress disorder (PTSD), depression, and anxiety. The meta-analysis also found that these interventions were associated with improvements in overall well-being, including decreased emotional reactivity and increased mindfulness.

Another study conducted in 2019 examined the effectiveness of mindfulness-based interventions in treating childhood trauma specifically. The study included 58 children and adolescents who had experienced trauma and found that those who received mindfulness-based interventions had significant reductions in symptoms of anxiety and depression, as well as improvements in overall well-being.

Benefits of Mindfulness-Based Therapies for Childhood Trauma

Mindfulness-based therapies have several potential benefits for individuals with childhood trauma, including:

- **Increased Self-Awareness:** Mindfulness-based therapies can help individuals with childhood trauma to develop a greater sense of self-awareness, allowing them to better understand their emotions and thought patterns.

- **Improved Emotional Regulation:** Mindfulness-based therapies can help individuals to regulate their emotions, allowing them to respond to difficult situations in a more adaptive way.

- **Reduced Anxiety and Depression:** Mindfulness-based therapies have been shown to be effective in reducing symptoms of anxiety and depression, which are common in individuals with childhood trauma.

- **Improved Overall Well-Being:** Mindfulness-based therapies can help individuals with childhood trauma to feel more connected to themselves and others, leading to an overall sense of well-being.

- **Reduced Stress:** Childhood trauma can cause chronic stress, which can have negative effects on mental and physical health. Mindfulness-based therapies can help individuals to reduce their stress levels, leading to improved health outcomes.

- **Improved Relationships:** Mindfulness-based therapies can help individuals with childhood trauma to develop more positive relationships with themselves and others, leading to improved social support and better overall well-being.

- **Improved Cognitive Functioning:** Childhood trauma can have negative effects on cognitive functioning, including memory and attention. Mindfulness-based therapies can help individuals to improve their cognitive functioning, leading to better academic and occupational outcomes.

- **Increased Resilience:** Childhood trauma can make individuals more vulnerable to future stressors. Mindfulness-based therapies can help individuals to develop resilience, allowing them to better cope with future challenges.

- **Reduced Reliance on Medications:** Mindfulness-based therapies can be a non-pharmacological approach to treating trauma-related symptoms, reducing the need for medications that can have negative side effects.

Mindfulness-based therapies have shown promise in helping individuals with trauma-related symptoms to manage their emotions, decrease anxiety and depression, and improve their overall well-being. There are several mindfulness-based therapies that have been developed to treat trauma-related symptoms, including Mindfulness-Based Stress Reduction (MBSR), Mindfulness-Based Cognitive Therapy (MBCT), and Mindfulness-Oriented Recovery Enhancement (MORE). Studies have found that these therapies are effective in reducing symptoms of PTSD, depression, and anxiety, and can improve overall well-being. Mindfulness-based therapies have several potential benefits for individuals with childhood trauma, including increased self-awareness, improved emotional regulation, reduced anxiety and depression, improved overall well-being, and increased resilience.

PSYCHODYNAMIC THERAPY FOR CHILDHOOD TRAUMA

Psychodynamic therapy is a form of therapy that emphasizes the role of unconscious thoughts and feelings in shaping behavior and relationships. This therapy approach is often used to help individuals who have experienced childhood trauma. Childhood trauma can take many forms, including physical abuse, sexual abuse, emotional abuse, neglect, or witnessing violence. Trauma can have long-lasting effects on a person's mental health and wellbeing, including anxiety, depression, and post-traumatic stress disorder (PTSD). Psychodynamic therapy aims to help individuals understand how their past experiences shape their current thoughts, feelings, and behaviors, and to work through any unresolved emotional conflicts.

Understanding Childhood Trauma

Before delving into psychodynamic therapy, it is important to understand what childhood trauma is and how it can affect individuals. Childhood trauma can be defined as any experience that threatens a child's physical or emotional wellbeing. Traumatic events can be a one-time occurrence or can happen repeatedly, such as in cases of ongoing abuse or neglect. Childhood trauma can have both immediate and long-term effects on an individual's mental and physical health.

The impact of childhood trauma can vary widely from person to person. Some individuals may experience no lasting effects, while others may develop mental health disorders, such as anxiety or depression, or physical health problems, such as chronic pain or cardiovascular disease. Childhood trauma can also affect an individual's ability to form healthy relationships, trust others, and regulate emotions.

Psychodynamic Therapy

This therapy approach is based on the idea that early childhood experiences shape a person's personality and behavior in adulthood. In the case of childhood trauma, psychodynamic therapy aims to help individuals identify and work through any unresolved emotional conflicts that may have stemmed from their traumatic experiences.

Psychodynamic therapy typically involves weekly sessions with a therapist, who will help the individual explore their thoughts, emotions, and behaviors in a safe and supportive environment. The therapist will use a variety of techniques to help the individual gain insight into their unconscious thoughts and feelings, including free association, dream analysis, and transference.

Free association involves the individual saying whatever comes to mind, without censoring or editing their thoughts. The therapist will listen carefully and help the individual explore any underlying emotions or memories that may be contributing to their current difficulties.

Dream analysis involves exploring the content of the individual's dreams to uncover any unconscious thoughts or feelings that may be influencing their behavior.

Transference occurs when the individual unconsciously projects their feelings about a significant person from their past onto the therapist. This can provide valuable insight into the individual's past experiences and help them work through any unresolved emotional conflicts.

During psychodynamic therapy, the therapist will also work with the individual to identify patterns of behavior or relationships that may be linked to their childhood trauma. By gaining insight into these patterns, the individual can learn to recognize and change them, leading to improved mental health and wellbeing.

Effectiveness of Psychodynamic Therapy for Childhood Trauma

Research has shown that psychodynamic therapy can be effective in treating childhood trauma. A 2016 review of 11 studies found that psychodynamic therapy was associated with significant improvements in symptoms of PTSD, depression, and anxiety in individuals with a history of childhood trauma.

The study also found that psychodynamic therapy was associated with improvements in self-esteem and interpersonal relationships.

One of the strengths of psychodynamic therapy is its focus on uncovering underlying emotional conflicts that may be contributing to an individual's difficulties. By gaining insight into these conflicts, individuals can develop a better understanding of their behavior and emotions, which can lead to long-lasting improvements in mental health and wellbeing.

It is important to note that psychodynamic therapy is typically a long-term therapy approach that may require several months or even years of weekly sessions

Summarized benefits of psychodynamic therapy:

- **Increased self-awareness**: By exploring unconscious thoughts and feelings, individuals can gain a better understanding of their behavior and emotions.
- **Improved relationships**: By identifying patterns of behavior and relationships, individuals can learn to recognize and change them, leading to improved interpersonal relationships.

- **Better emotional regulation**: By working through unresolved emotional conflicts, individuals can learn to regulate their emotions and manage stress more effectively.

- **Improved coping skills**: By gaining insight into their behavior and emotions, individuals can develop better coping skills and strategies to deal with difficult situations.

- **Treatment of mental health disorders:** Psychodynamic therapy has been shown to be effective in treating a range of mental health disorders, including depression, anxiety, and PTSD.

- **Long-lasting improvements:** The insights gained through psychodynamic therapy can lead to long-lasting improvements in mental health and wellbeing.

It is important to note that the benefits of psychodynamic therapy may vary from person to person and may require several months or even years of weekly sessions.

NARRATIVE THERAPY FOR CHILDHOOD TRAUMA

Narrative therapy is a type of psychotherapy that is based on the premise that people have unique stories and experiences that shape their identity and behavior. Narrative therapy for childhood trauma focuses on helping children to understand and reinterpret their traumatic experiences in a way that allows them to regain a sense of agency and control over their lives. In this article, we will explore the principles and techniques of narrative therapy for childhood trauma in detail.

Narrative Therapy Principles

Narrative therapy is based on several principles that guide the therapeutic process. These principles are:

- **Respect for the client's experience:** The therapist respects the client's experience and perspective and helps the client to explore and understand their experiences in a way that is meaningful to them.
- **Externalization:** Narrative therapy externalizes problems by separating the problem from the person. The problem is viewed as a separate entity that can be examined and addressed.

- **Deconstruction:** Narrative therapy deconstructs dominant cultural narratives and helps clients to create new narratives that better reflect their experiences.

- **Re-authoring:** Narrative therapy involves the process of re-authoring or rewriting a client's story to reflect a more positive and empowering view of themselves.

- **Collaborative approach**: Narrative therapy is a collaborative process that involves a partnership between the therapist and the client. The therapist helps the client to explore and understand their experiences while empowering them to take control of their lives.

Narrative Therapy Techniques

Narrative therapy uses a variety of techniques to help children to externalize and reauthor their experiences. These techniques include:

- **Creating a safe and supportive environment**: The therapist creates a safe and supportive environment where the child feels comfortable sharing their experiences.

- **Exploring the child's experience:** The therapist helps the child to explore their experience in a way that is meaningful to them. This may involve asking open-ended questions, using metaphors, and exploring the emotions associated with the experience.

- **Externalizing the problem:** The therapist helps the child to externalize the problem by separating the problem from the child. This may involve using a metaphor, such as viewing the problem as a monster or a dragon.

- **Deconstructing dominant cultural narratives:** The therapist helps the child to deconstruct dominant cultural narratives that may be contributing to their feelings of shame or helplessness. For example, a child who has experienced abuse may believe that they are to blame for the abuse, and the therapist may help the child to understand that the abuse was not their fault.

- **Reauthoring the child's story:** The therapist helps the child to reauthor their story by creating a new, more positive narrative that better reflects their experiences. This may involve helping the child to identify their strengths, resilience, and accomplishments.

- **Using creative expression:** Narrative therapy may involve using creative expression to help the child to externalize and explore their experiences. This may involve using art, music, or play therapy.

- **Empowering the child:** The therapist empowers the child by helping them to regain a sense of agency and control over their lives. This may involve helping the child to identify their goals and develop strategies for achieving them.

Benefits of Narrative Therapy for Childhood Trauma

Narrative therapy for childhood trauma has several benefits. These benefits include:

- **Increased self-esteem and self-worth:** Narrative therapy helps children to create a new, more positive narrative about themselves that reflects their true self and strength.

- **Increased resilience:** Narrative therapy helps children to develop resilience by helping them to identify and build on their strengths and resources. This can help children to cope with future challenges and setbacks.

- **Improved emotional regulation:** Narrative therapy helps children to identify and express their emotions in a healthy way. This can help children to develop better emotional regulation skills and reduce the likelihood of engaging in maladaptive coping behaviors such as substance abuse or self-harm.

- **Improved relationships:** Narrative therapy can improve children's relationships by helping them to understand and communicate their experiences and emotions to others. This can help children to develop stronger, more supportive relationships with family, friends, and other important people in their lives.

- **Reduced symptoms of trauma:** Narrative therapy can help to reduce the symptoms of trauma such as anxiety, depression, and PTSD. By externalizing and reauthoring their traumatic experiences, children can gain a greater sense of control over their lives and reduce the impact of the trauma on their mental health.

- **Increased sense of agency**: Narrative therapy helps children to regain a sense of agency and control over their lives. By helping children to identify their goals and develop strategies for achieving them, narrative therapy can help children to feel more empowered and in control of their lives.

- **Improved academic performance:** Narrative therapy can improve children's academic performance by reducing the impact of trauma on their cognitive and emotional functioning. By helping children to regulate their emotions and improve their self-esteem, narrative therapy can help children to perform better in school and achieve their academic goals.

Overall, narrative therapy is a powerful and effective tool for helping children to cope with and overcome the effects of childhood trauma. By helping children to externalize and re-author their experiences, narrative therapy can help children to regain a sense of control over their lives and develop the skills and resources they need to thrive.

ART THERAPY FOR CHILDHOOD TRAUMA

Art therapy is a psychotherapeutic intervention that incorporates the use of creative expression, such as drawing, painting, and sculpting, to help individuals improve their mental and emotional well-being. Art therapy has been found to be an effective treatment for a variety of mental health issues, including childhood trauma. Childhood trauma is a significant risk factor for developing mental health problems in adulthood, such as anxiety, depression, and post-traumatic stress disorder (PTSD). Art therapy can be a powerful tool in helping children process and heal from their trauma.

The Role of the Art Therapist

Art therapists are trained mental health professionals who use art as a therapeutic tool. Art therapists work with children to create a safe and supportive environment where the child can explore their emotions and feelings through creative expression. The art therapist helps the child process their artwork, guiding them to identify and express their emotions and thoughts.

Art Therapy Techniques for Childhood Trauma

- **Drawing and Painting:** Drawing and painting are common art therapy techniques used for children who have experienced trauma. These techniques allow the child to express their emotions and feelings in a nonverbal way. The art therapist may ask the child to draw or paint their feelings, or to create a picture of their trauma.

- **Collage:** Collage is another art therapy technique that can be helpful for children who have experienced trauma. Collage involves creating a picture using various materials such as paper, magazines, and photographs. The child can use these materials to create a visual representation of their trauma or to express their feelings in a nonverbal way.

- **Sculpting:** Sculpting is another art therapy technique that can be helpful for children who have experienced trauma. Sculpting involves using various materials such as clay or play dough to create a three-dimensional object. The child can use this technique to create a representation of their trauma or to express their emotions and feelings.

Benefits of Art Therapy for Childhood Trauma

- **Increased Self-Awareness:** Art therapy can help individuals gain a better understanding of their emotions and thoughts. Creating art can be a way for individuals to explore and express their inner experiences, allowing them to develop a deeper sense of self-awareness.

- **Improved Communication:** Art therapy can help individuals who struggle with verbal communication express themselves in a nonverbal way. Creating art can be a way for individuals to communicate their emotions and experiences to others in a visual and tangible way.

- **Enhanced Problem-Solving Skills:** Creating art can require problem-solving skills, such as deciding which materials to use or how to structure a piece. Art therapy can help individuals develop these skills, which can be applied to other areas of their lives.

- **Improved Emotional Regulation:** Art therapy can help children regulate their emotions and exercise an appreciable level of control over their emotions.

- **Stress Reduction:** Creating art can be a calming and relaxing activity, which can help individuals reduce stress and anxiety. Art therapy can provide a safe and supportive environment for individuals to process their emotions and find a sense of calm.

- **Increased Self-Esteem:** Creating art can be a way for individuals to express themselves creatively and feel a sense of accomplishment. Art therapy can help individuals develop a sense of self-worth and confidence in their abilities.

- **Trauma Recovery:** As mentioned earlier, art therapy can be particularly helpful for individuals who have experienced trauma. Creating art can provide a safe and supportive outlet for individuals to process their trauma and develop coping skills.

- **Improved Physical Health:** Creating art can be a physically engaging activity that can help individuals develop fine motor skills and hand-eye coordination. This can be particularly beneficial for individuals with physical disabilities or conditions that affect their motor skills.

Overall, art therapy can be a powerful tool for improving mental and emotional well-being, as well as physical health. The benefits of art therapy can be experienced by individuals of all ages and backgrounds, and can be particularly helpful for those who have experienced trauma or struggle with verbal communication.

YOGA THERAPY FOR CHILDHOOD TRAUMA

Yoga therapy has emerged as an effective complementary treatment option for children who have experienced trauma. Childhood trauma, whether physical, emotional or psychological, can have long-lasting effects on a child's development, behavior and mental health. Yoga therapy offers a holistic approach that can help children process and manage their trauma, while also improving their overall health and wellbeing.

Yoga therapy uses physical postures, breathing exercises, meditation, and mindfulness to promote healing and wellbeing. Yoga has been shown to reduce stress, anxiety, and depression, and improve mood, cognitive function, and physical health. Yoga therapy is especially beneficial for children who have experienced trauma, as it can help them regulate their emotions, improve their self-awareness, and develop healthy coping skills.

Yoga therapy can be adapted to meet the needs of children of all ages and abilities, and can be practiced individually or in group settings. A typical yoga therapy session for children may include a combination of physical postures, breathing exercises, and relaxation techniques, along with guided imagery and visualization.

Benefits of Yoga Therapy for Childhood Trauma

Yoga therapy offers a range of benefits for children who have experienced trauma, including:

- **Stress reduction:** Yoga therapy helps children regulate their stress response, by activating the parasympathetic nervous system, which induces a state of relaxation and calmness.

- **Improved self-awareness:** Yoga therapy helps children become more aware of their body, mind, and emotions, and develop a greater sense of self-awareness and self-compassion.

- **Emotional regulation:** Yoga therapy teaches children to regulate their emotions and manage difficult feelings, such as anxiety, anger, and fear, through breathing techniques and mindfulness practices.

- **Increased resilience:** Yoga therapy helps children build resilience, by developing their coping skills, and promoting a sense of self-efficacy and empowerment.

- **Improved physical health:** Yoga therapy helps children improve their physical health, by promoting flexibility, strength, and balance, and reducing symptoms of chronic pain and illness.

Yoga Therapy Techniques for Childhood Trauma

- **Physical postures (asanas):** Yoga therapy uses a range of physical postures that are designed to improve strength, flexibility, balance, and coordination. These postures can be adapted to meet the needs of children of all ages and abilities.

- **Breathing exercises (pranayama):** Yoga therapy uses a range of breathing exercises that are designed to regulate the breath, calm the mind, and reduce stress and anxiety. Children can learn to use these techniques to manage their emotions and improve their mental wellbeing.

- **Mindfulness and meditation:** Yoga therapy uses mindfulness and meditation techniques that are designed to promote self-awareness, relaxation, and mental clarity. These techniques can help children manage their thoughts and emotions, and improve their overall mental health.

- **Guided visualization:** Yoga therapy uses guided visualization techniques that are designed to help children process and manage their trauma. These techniques can help children develop a sense of safety and security, and improve their overall wellbeing.

- **Yoga nidra:** Yoga nidra is a form of deep relaxation that is designed to promote physical, mental, and emotional relaxation. This technique can help children reduce stress, improve sleep, and promote healing and recovery.

There are several case studies that demonstrate the effectiveness of yoga

Case Study 1: Yoga Therapy for Child Survivors of Hurricane Katrina

A study published in the International Journal of Yoga Therapy examined the effects of yoga therapy on child survivors of Hurricane Katrina, a catastrophic natural disaster that occurred in 2005. The study involved 22 children, ages 6 to 12, who were living in temporary housing at the time of the study. The children participated in a 12-week yoga therapy program that included physical postures, breathing exercises, relaxation techniques, and meditation.

The study found that the children who participated in the yoga therapy program showed significant improvements in their overall wellbeing, including reduced symptoms of anxiety and depression, improved self-esteem, and increased resilience. The researchers concluded that yoga therapy can be an effective treatment option for child survivors of traumatic events, such as natural disasters.

Case Study 2: Yoga Therapy for Child Refugees

A study published in the Journal of Traumatic Stress examined the effects of yoga therapy on child refugees who had experienced trauma, including war, violence, and displacement. The study involved 16 child refugees, ages 9 to 12, who were living in a refugee camp at the time of the study. The children participated in a 6-week yoga therapy program that included physical postures, breathing exercises, and relaxation techniques.

The study found that the children who participated in the yoga therapy program showed significant improvements in their overall wellbeing, including reduced symptoms of anxiety and depression, improved sleep quality, and increased resilience. The researchers concluded that yoga therapy can be an effective treatment option for child refugees who have experienced trauma.

Case Study 3: Yoga Therapy for Child Victims of Sexual Abuse

A study published in the Journal of Child Sexual Abuse examined the effects of yoga therapy on child victims of sexual abuse. The study involved 42 children, ages 8 to 12, who had experienced sexual abuse and were receiving therapy at a community mental health center. The children participated in a 12-week yoga therapy program that included physical postures, breathing exercises, relaxation techniques, and meditation.

The study found that the children who participated in the yoga therapy program showed significant improvements in their overall wellbeing, including reduced symptoms of anxiety and depression, improved self-esteem, and increased resilience. The researchers concluded that yoga therapy can be an effective complementary treatment option for child victims of sexual abuse, in addition to traditional therapy.

Overall, these case studies demonstrate the effectiveness of yoga therapy for childhood trauma. Yoga therapy can provide children with a holistic approach to healing and wellbeing, and can help them manage the emotional and psychological effects of trauma.

GROUP THERAPY FOR CHILDHOOD TRAUMA

Group therapy is a well-established treatment option for childhood trauma, providing a supportive and collaborative environment for individuals to explore their experiences and work towards healing. Here, I will talk about group therapy for childhood trauma in detail, including its benefits, process, and effectiveness.

Benefits of Group Therapy for Childhood Trauma

Group therapy for childhood trauma provides many benefits to individuals who have experienced trauma. Some of these benefits include:

- **Support from Peers:** Group therapy allows individuals to connect with others who have experienced similar traumatic events. This can be helpful in providing a sense of validation and understanding, which is often difficult to find in other settings.

- **A Safe and Confidential Environment:** Group therapy provides a safe and confidential environment where individuals can share their experiences without fear of judgment or reprisal.

- **Learning from Others:** Group therapy allows individuals to learn from others who have experienced similar traumatic events. This can be helpful in gaining new insights and perspectives, as well as learning coping strategies that have worked for others.

- **Developing Coping Skills:** Group therapy provides an opportunity for individuals to develop coping skills that can help them manage their emotions and reactions to trauma triggers.

- **Building Resilience:** Group therapy can help individuals build resilience and develop a sense of empowerment in their healing journey.

Process of Group Therapy for Childhood Trauma

The process of group therapy for childhood trauma typically involves the following steps:

- **Group Formation:** The first step in group therapy for childhood trauma is forming the group. This typically involves recruiting individuals who have experienced similar traumatic events and are at a similar stage in their healing journey.

- **Assessment:** Once the group is formed, each individual undergoes an assessment to determine their specific needs and goals for therapy.

- **Group Sessions:** Group sessions typically last for 60 to 90 minutes and are held on a regular basis (e.g. weekly or bi-weekly). During these sessions, individuals share their experiences and feelings, and the group provides support and feedback.

- **Facilitator Role:** The facilitator plays a crucial role in group therapy for childhood trauma, providing guidance and support to the group. The facilitator may also introduce specific exercises or activities to help individuals develop coping skills and build resilience.

- **Group Dynamics:** The dynamics of the group are also important in group therapy for childhood trauma. As the group progresses, individuals may develop closer connections with certain members, and conflicts may arise. The facilitator plays a crucial role in managing these dynamics and ensuring that the group remains a safe and supportive environment.

Effectiveness of Group Therapy for Childhood Trauma

Research has shown that group therapy can be an effective treatment option for childhood trauma. A meta-analysis of 32 studies found that group therapy was associated with significant reductions in symptoms of post-traumatic stress disorder (PTSD), depression, and anxiety in individuals who have experienced childhood trauma (Cohen et al., 2010).

Other studies have also found that group therapy can improve social functioning, reduce feelings of isolation and shame, and improve overall quality of life for individuals who have experienced childhood trauma.

One of the key advantages of group therapy for childhood trauma is that it provides a supportive and collaborative environment that can be difficult to find in other settings. This environment can help individuals feel less isolated and more empowered in their healing journey, which can contribute to better treatment outcomes.

Group therapy for childhood trauma is a valuable treatment option for individuals who have experienced traumatic events in their childhood. It provides a supportive and collaborative environment where individuals can connect with others who have had similar experiences, develop

COPING STRATEGIES FOR TRAUMA

Coping strategies can help these individuals manage their symptoms and improve their quality of life.

There are many coping strategies that victims of childhood trauma can use to manage their symptoms. These strategies can be divided into four categories: physical, cognitive, emotional, and behavioral.

Physical Coping Strategies

Physical coping strategies involve activities that help victims of childhood trauma reduce physical symptoms of stress and anxiety. These strategies include:

- **Exercise** - Exercise can help reduce anxiety and depression by releasing endorphins, which are natural mood-boosters. Victims of childhood trauma can engage in physical activities like jogging, walking, cycling, swimming, or practicing yoga. These activities help to regulate breathing and decrease stress.
- **Sleep** - Victims of childhood trauma can adopt a sleep routine to ensure that they get enough sleep. This includes maintaining a regular sleep schedule, avoiding caffeine and electronic devices before bedtime, and creating a comfortable sleep environment.
- **Diet** - Eating a healthy diet can help reduce stress and anxiety. Victims of childhood trauma should avoid processed foods, sugary foods, and alcohol, which can exacerbate stress and anxiety symptoms. Instead, they

should eat a diet rich in fruits, vegetables, whole grains, and lean proteins.

- **Relaxation Techniques** – a victim of childhood trauma can apply some relaxation techniques which includes meditation, deep breathing and others these techniques regularly to help manage their symptoms.

Cognitive Coping Strategies

Cognitive coping strategies involve changing the way victims of childhood trauma think about their experiences. These strategies include:

- **Self-Talk** - Victims of childhood trauma can use positive self-talk to change their negative thoughts into positive ones. This involves replacing negative thoughts with positive affirmations, such as "I am strong" or "I am worthy."

- **Cognitive Reframing** - Cognitive reframing involves looking at a situation from a different perspective. Victims of childhood trauma can reframe their negative thoughts by asking themselves questions like, "Is this thought realistic?" or "Is there another way to look at this situation?"

- **Mindfulness** - Victims of childhood trauma can practice mindfulness by focusing on their breathing, paying attention to their senses, and being aware of their thoughts and feelings.
- **Gratitude** -. Victims of childhood trauma can keep a gratitude journal or list three things they are grateful for each day. Learn to focus on the positive aspects of life. This can help realign their focus from harmful negative thoughts to positive ones.

Emotional Coping Strategies

Emotional coping strategies involve managing and regulating one's emotions. These strategies include:

- **Emotional Awareness** - Victims of childhood trauma can become more aware of their emotions by identifying their triggers and recognizing their emotional responses. This can help them regulate their emotions more effectively.
- **Emotional Expression** - Expressing emotions can help victims of childhood trauma cope with their experiences. This can involve talking to a therapist, a trusted friend, or a support group. Victims can also use art or writing as a way to express their emotions.

- **Self-Compassion** - Victims of childhood trauma can practice self-compassion by treating themselves with kindness and understanding. This involves being patient with oneself and recognizing that healing takes time.

- **Distraction** - Distraction techniques can help victims of childhood trauma cope with difficult emotions. This can involve engaging in activities like watching a movie, reading a book, or listening to music.

Seek Professional Help

One of the most important coping strategies for individuals who have experienced childhood trauma is to seek professional help. A mental health professional can help a person understand and process their trauma in a safe and supportive environment. Therapy can provide individuals with coping skills, such as relaxation techniques that can help them manage anxiety and other symptoms related to trauma.

Practice Self-Care

Self-care is an essential aspect of coping with childhood trauma. Engaging in activities that promote self-care can help individuals manage stress and improve their mental health.

Some self-care practices include exercise, healthy eating, getting enough sleep, spending time in nature, and engaging in hobbies or activities that bring joy.

Develop a Support System

Having a support system is crucial when coping with childhood trauma. A support system can include family, friends, and mental health professionals. Individuals who have experienced childhood trauma may also benefit from joining a support group with other individuals who have had similar experiences. This can help in providing a supportive environment which can help in the recovery of victims of childhood trauma.

Learn Stress Management Techniques

Stress management techniques can help individuals cope with the physical and emotional symptoms of trauma. Techniques such as deep breathing, progressive muscle relaxation, and visualization can help individuals manage anxiety and other symptoms related to trauma.

Identify Triggers

Triggers are events or situations that can cause a person to experience negative emotions or feelings related to their trauma. Identifying triggers can help individuals avoid situations that may cause them distress or trigger memories of their trauma.

Set Boundaries

Setting boundaries is an important aspect of coping with childhood trauma. Individuals who have experienced trauma may struggle with setting boundaries in their relationships. Setting boundaries can help individuals feel safe and in control of their interactions with others.

Practice Forgiveness

Forgiveness is an important aspect of healing from childhood trauma. Forgiving oneself and others can help individuals let go of anger and resentment and move forward in their healing process.

Engage in Creative Expression

Engaging in creative expression can be a powerful way for individuals to cope with childhood trauma. Writing, painting, and other forms of creative expression can help individuals express their emotions and process their trauma in a healthy and constructive way.

Take Small Steps

Healing from childhood trauma is a process that takes time. Individuals who have experienced trauma should take small steps towards healing and not try to rush the process. It is essential to be patient and compassionate with oneself during the healing process.

Develop Coping Strategies

Developing coping strategies can help individuals manage their emotions and symptoms related to trauma. Coping strategies may include self-care practices, stress management techniques, mindfulness, and other techniques that have been helpful in managing symptoms.

Practice Gratitude

Practicing gratitude can help individuals focus on positive aspects of their life and increase their overall sense of well-being. Individuals who have experienced trauma may find it challenging to focus on positive aspects of their life. Practicing gratitude can help shift their focus towards positive aspects of their life.

Develop a Safety Plan

Individuals who have experienced childhood trauma may struggle with feelings of safety and security. Developing a safety plan can help individuals feel more in control.

ROLE OF FAMILY IN TRAUMA

The effects of childhood trauma can be long-lasting, affecting not only the child's mental health but also their physical and emotional wellbeing as they grow into adulthood. In this context, the role of parents, guardians, and siblings is crucial in helping victims of childhood trauma to heal and recover.

1. **Acknowledge the Trauma**

The first step in helping a child who has experienced trauma is to acknowledge what has happened to them. Parents, guardians, and siblings need to understand and accept that the child has experienced something that was beyond their control and was deeply distressing. Acknowledging the trauma is important because it helps the child to feel heard, validated, and understood. It also creates a safe space for the child to express their feelings and emotions.

2. **Provide Emotional Support**

Children who have experienced trauma may feel isolated, scared, and confused. Parents, guardians, and siblings can provide emotional support by listening to the child, validating their feelings, and offering comfort and reassurance. It is important to create a safe and supportive environment for the child where they can express themselves freely without fear of judgment or criticism.

3. **Seek Professional Help**

While parents, guardians, and siblings can provide emotional support, it is important to seek professional help for the child. Trauma can have long-lasting effects on a child's mental health, and it is important to get the child the help they need to heal and recover. Professional help can come in the form of therapy, counseling, or other types of mental health support.

4. **Create a Routine**

Children who have experienced trauma may feel like they have lost control over their lives. Creating a routine can help the child feel more in control and secure. The routine can include regular mealtimes, bedtime, and other daily activities. This can help the child feel more stable and secure.

5. **Encourage Self-Care**

Self-care is essential for everyone, but it is especially important for children who have experienced trauma. Parents, guardians, and siblings can encourage the child to engage in self-care activities such as exercise, meditation, reading, or other activities that the child enjoys. This can help the child to relax, reduce stress, and feel more positive.

6. **Build Trust**

Children who have experienced trauma may struggle with trust issues. Building trust is important in helping the child feel safe and secure. Parents, guardians, and siblings can build trust by being reliable, keeping their promises, and being consistent in their actions.

7. **Encourage Positive Relationships**

Positive relationships are important for a child's mental health and wellbeing. Parents, guardians, and siblings can encourage the child to develop positive relationships with friends, family members, or other supportive adults. This can help the child feel more connected and supported.

8. **Practice Patience**

Healing from childhood trauma can take time. Parents, guardians, and siblings need to practice patience and understand that healing is a process. It is important not to rush the child or put pressure on them to heal quickly. Instead, it is important to provide consistent support and encouragement throughout the healing process.

9. **Foster a Positive Environment**

Creating a positive environment is essential for a child's mental health and wellbeing. Parents, guardians, and siblings can foster a positive environment by promoting positivity, creating a safe and comfortable space, and encouraging the child to engage in activities that they enjoy. This can help the child feel more positive and reduce stress.

10. **Be Available**

Children who have experienced trauma may need extra support and attention.

The effects of childhood trauma in a person's life can be long lasting. It can lead to emotional and psychological problems, affect social relationships, and interfere with daily functioning.

Victims of childhood trauma require help and support to overcome the negative effects of their experiences. This is where parents, guardians, and siblings can play a crucial role in helping the victim heal from their trauma.

The Role of Parents

Parents are often the primary caregivers and have a significant influence on a child's development. In cases where a child has experienced trauma, parents play a crucial role in helping them heal and recover some ways parents can help a victim includes:

1. **Be Supportive:** The first step is to provide emotional support and create a safe environment where the child feels comfortable sharing their feelings. It's essential to listen actively without judgment and validate their emotions.
2. **Seek Professional Help:** Parents should seek professional help, such as a therapist or counselor, to help their child cope with the trauma. A professional can help the child understand their feelings, develop coping mechanisms, and work through the trauma.
3. **Create a Routine:** Children benefit from having a routine as it provides a sense of stability and

predictability. Parents can create a daily schedule that includes activities, chores, and time for relaxation and self-care.

4. **Model Healthy Coping Strategies:** Parents should model healthy coping strategies such as exercise, mindfulness, and relaxation techniques. This will teach the child positive ways to manage their emotions and reduce stress.

5. **Advocate for the Child:** Parents should advocate for their child and ensure that they receive the support and resources they need. This includes working with schools, medical professionals, and community resources to provide the child with the necessary assistance.

The Role of Guardians:

Guardians are responsible for the welfare and care of a child who is not their own. In cases where a child has experienced trauma, guardians can play a significant role in helping the child heal and recover. Here are some ways guardians can help:

1. **Build Trust:** Building trust is essential in helping a child heal from trauma. Guardians should create a safe

and secure environment and establish a trusting relationship with the child.

2. **Provide Emotional Support:** Guardians should provide emotional support and create a space where the child feels comfortable sharing their feelings. It's essential to listen actively without judgment and validate their emotions.

3. **Seek Professional Help:** Guardians should seek professional help, such as a therapist or counselor, this will help the child in your care heal and leave all of the pains behind.

The Role of Siblings:

Siblings can play a crucial role in helping a child heal from trauma. Siblings may have experienced similar traumatic events, and their support can be particularly valuable in these situations. Here are some ways siblings can help:

1. **Be Supportive:** Siblings can be supportive by listening to the child's feelings and validating their emotions. It's essential to create a safe space where the child feels comfortable sharing their experiences.

2. **Provide Emotional Support:** Siblings can provide emotional support by being there for the child and

offering comfort and reassurance. They can also provide a sense of stability and predictability by engaging in activities together.

3. **Seek Professional Help:** Siblings can encourage the child to seek professional help, such as a therapist or counselor, to help them cope

4. **Offer Distraction:** Siblings can offer a distraction from the trauma by engaging in fun and enjoyable activities together. This can help the child take their mind off their experiences and provide a sense of normalcy.

5. **Be Patient:** It's important for siblings to be patient and understanding as the child works through their trauma. Healing from trauma is a process that takes time, and it's essential to be supportive throughout the journey.

6. **Educate Themselves:** Siblings can educate themselves about the effects of trauma and how to support someone who has experienced it. This can help them better understand their sibling's experiences and how they can help.

7. **Be a Role Model:** Siblings can be a positive role model for the child by modeling healthy coping mechanisms and positive behaviors. This can help the

child develop healthy habits and strategies for managing their emotions.

Childhood trauma can have a significant impact on a person's life, but with the right support, victims can heal and recover. Parents, guardians, and siblings can play a crucial role in helping the child through their trauma. It's essential to provide emotional support, seek professional help, create a routine, advocate for the child, and be patient throughout the healing process. By working together, we can help victims of childhood trauma heal and move forward with their lives.

GOALS AFTER CHILDHOOD TRAUMA

Setting goals and moving forward in the case of childhood trauma is a very important step in overcoming childhood trauma. It is important because it will provide for you a form of direction which will lead you away from the demeaning feelings that will often arise from the impacts of childhood trauma.

The first step towards setting goals and moving forward in the case of childhood trauma is to understand the impact it has had on your life. Childhood trauma can manifest in many ways, including anxiety, depression, low self-esteem, relationship problems, and substance abuse. By understanding the impact of childhood trauma on your life, you can develop a greater sense of self-awareness, which is essential to set achievable goals. Some steps that will help in this process includes:

Seeking professional help:

Childhood trauma can be challenging to overcome, and it is essential to seek professional help. A therapist can help you understand the impact of childhood trauma on your life, develop coping strategies, and set achievable goals. A therapist can also provide you with tools to manage the challenges you may face when working towards your goals.

Setting small, achievable goals:

Setting small, achievable goals is crucial when you are dealing with childhood trauma. The process of setting goals can be overwhelming, and setting small, achievable goals can help you build confidence and self-esteem. Start with simple goals like going for a walk every day or reading a chapter of a book. As you achieve these goals, you can gradually increase the complexity and scope of your goals.

Breaking down your goals into manageable steps:

Breaking down your goals into manageable steps is an effective way to achieve your goals. For example, if your goal is to complete a college degree, break it down into manageable steps like researching schools, applying for financial aid, registering for classes, and attending lectures. Breaking down your goals into manageable steps can help you stay focused and motivated.

Developing a support network:

Developing a support network is essential when you are dealing with childhood trauma. Your support network can include friends, family members, and professionals like therapists and support groups. Your support network can provide you with emotional support, encouragement, and motivation when you are working towards your goals.

Practicing self-care:

Self-care is essential when you are dealing with childhood trauma. Self-care activities like meditation, yoga, and exercise can help you reduce stress and anxiety, improve your mental and physical health, and increase your sense of self-worth.

Practicing self-care can also help you stay focused and motivated when you are working towards your goals.

Being patient and kind to yourself:

Dealing with childhood trauma can be challenging, and it is essential to be patient and kind to yourself. There may be setbacks and obstacles along the way, and it is important to acknowledge and accept them without judgment. Be gentle with yourself and celebrate your successes, no matter how small.

Celebrating your successes:

Celebrating your successes is an essential part of setting goals and moving forward in the case of childhood trauma. Celebrate your successes, no matter how small. Celebrating your successes can help you stay motivated and focused on achieving your goals.

Practicing mindfulness:

Practicing mindfulness can help you reduce stress and anxiety, improve your mental and physical health, and increase your sense of self-awareness. Mindfulness can also help you stay focused and motivated when you are working towards your goals.

Using affirmations:

Affirmations are positive statements that you repeat to yourself to reinforce positive beliefs about yourself. Using affirmations can help you overcome negative self-talk, increase your self-esteem, and stay motivated when you are working towards your goals. Examples of affirm

Identifying your values:

Identifying your values can help you set goals that align with your priorities and give your life meaning and purpose. This can help you set goals that are meaningful and fulfilling.

Learning to manage triggers:

Childhood trauma can create triggers that cause emotional and physical distress. Learning to manage triggers can help you stay focused and motivated when you are working towards your goals. You can learn coping strategies to manage triggers, such as deep breathing, visualization, and progressive muscle relaxation.

Practicing forgiveness:

Forgiveness can be a powerful tool when dealing with childhood trauma. Forgiveness is not about forgetting or condoning the past, but about letting go of anger and resentment that may be holding you back. Forgiveness can help you move forward and focus on the present and future.

Practicing gratitude:

Practicing gratitude can help you focus on the positive aspects of your life, even when dealing with childhood trauma. Take some time each day to reflect on the things you are grateful for, such as supportive friends, a comfortable home, or good health. Practicing gratitude can help you cultivate a positive outlook on life.

Setting boundaries:

Setting boundaries can help you protect your physical and emotional well-being when dealing with childhood trauma. This may involve setting limits on the amount of time you spend with certain people or in certain situations. Setting boundaries can help you feel empowered and in control of your life.

Using visualization:

Visualization involves creating mental images of achieving your goals. Visualization can help you stay motivated and focused on your goals, even when facing obstacles or setbacks. Take some time each day to visualize yourself achieving your goals, and imagine how you will feel when you accomplish them.

Practicing self-compassion:

Self-compassion involves treating yourself with kindness and understanding, rather than judgment and criticism. Self-compassion can help you overcome negative self-talk and increase your sense of self-worth. When working towards your goals, practice self-compassion by acknowledging your strengths and weaknesses, and treating yourself with kindness and patience.

Building resilience:

Building resilience can help you cope with the challenges of childhood trauma and achieve your goals. Resilience involves developing skills and strategies to overcome adversity and bounce back from setbacks. Building resilience can involve learning coping strategies, developing a positive outlook on life, and cultivating social support networks.

In conclusion, setting goals and moving forward in the case of childhood trauma can be challenging, but it is possible. By seeking professional help, setting small, achievable goals, developing a support network, practicing self-care, and using other strategies, you can overcome the impact of childhood trauma and achieve your goals. Remember to be patient and kind to yourself, celebrate your successes, and cultivate resilience and self-compassion along the way.

SUPPORTING SURVIVORS OF TRAUMA

(How victims of childhood trauma can help others)

Childhood trauma can have a profound and lasting impact on a person's life. Traumatic experiences during childhood can include physical, emotional, and sexual abuse, neglect, and exposure to violence. These experiences can have lasting effects on a person's physical, emotional, and mental health. However, survivors of childhood trauma can also use their experiences to help others who have gone through similar experiences. Some ways to achieve that includes:

- **Sharing One's Story:** One of the most powerful ways that survivors of childhood trauma can help others is by sharing their stories. There are several potential benefits to sharing one's story, including:

- **Breaking the silence:** Survivors of childhood trauma often feel alone and isolated in their experiences. By sharing their stories, they can help break the silence around these issues and create a sense of community among survivors.

- **Raising awareness**: Sharing one's story can also help raise awareness about childhood trauma and its impacts. This can help to reduce stigma and increase understanding about the needs of survivors.

- **Providing hope**: Survivors who have healed and moved forward in their lives can provide hope to others who are still struggling with their experiences. By sharing their stories of resilience and recovery, survivors can inspire others to seek help and make positive changes in their lives.

- **Creating change:** Survivors who speak out about their experiences can also be powerful advocates for change. By sharing their stories with policymakers, organizations, and communities, survivors can help to create policies and programs that better support survivors of childhood trauma.

Ways to Help Others

There are many ways that survivors of childhood trauma can help others. Some of these include:

- **Peer support:** Survivors can offer peer support to others who have gone through similar experiences. This can include participating in support groups, mentoring programs, or online communities.
- **Advocacy:** Survivors can also advocate for policies and programs that better support survivors of childhood trauma. This can include speaking with policymakers, participating in advocacy campaigns, or joining advocacy organizations.
- **Education:** Survivors can also help to educate others about childhood trauma and its impacts. This can include speaking at conferences or events, writing articles or blog posts, or creating educational materials.
- **Counseling and therapy:** Survivors who have gone through counseling or therapy can use their experiences to help others who are struggling with similar issues. This can include becoming a counselor or therapist

themselves, or volunteering with organizations that provide counseling services.

Strategies for Supporting Oneself

Supporting others can be rewarding, but it can also be emotionally challenging. Survivors of childhood trauma may need to take extra steps to support themselves while supporting others. Some strategies for self-care and support include:

- **Seeking support**: Survivors can seek support from friends, family, or professional counselors or therapists. Talking about one's experiences can be difficult, but it can also be helpful to have a supportive listener.
- **Setting boundaries:** Survivors may need to set boundaries to protect their own emotional wellbeing. This may include limiting the amount of time spent talking about their experiences, or avoiding triggering situations or conversations.
- **Practicing self-care:** Survivors can prioritize self-care activities that help them to feel calm, centered, and grounded. This can include exercise, meditation, creative expression, or spending time in nature.

- **Continuing personal growth:** Survivors can continue to work on their own personal growth and healing while helping others. This can include participating in therapy or counseling, practicing mindfulness, or pursuing hobbies or interests that bring joy and fulfillment.

- **Supporting advocacy efforts:** Survivors can support advocacy efforts by participating in marches, rallies, and other events that raise awareness about childhood trauma. They can also contribute financially to organizations that work to support survivors.

- **Volunteering with organizations:** Survivors can volunteer with organizations that provide support and services to survivors of childhood trauma. This can include volunteering at shelters, crisis hotlines, or organizations that provide counseling services.

- **Speaking at schools and universities:** Survivors can speak at schools and universities to educate students about the impact of childhood trauma. This can help students to understand the challenges that survivors face and to become advocates for change.

- **Mentoring programs:** Survivors can participate in mentoring programs that provide support to children who have experienced trauma. By sharing their experiences and providing guidance, survivors can help to support the healing and growth of younger generations.

- **Writing and publishing:** Survivors can write and publish books or articles that share their experiences and offer advice and support to others. This can include memoirs, self-help books, or articles in magazines or newspapers.

It is important to note that supporting others can be emotionally challenging for survivors of childhood trauma. It is important to prioritize self-care and support while supporting others. Survivors should also be mindful of their own emotional boundaries and needs and seek help when needed.

In conclusion, survivors of childhood trauma have a unique perspective and experience that can be invaluable in helping others who have gone through similar experiences. By sharing their stories, advocating for change, and providing support to others, survivors can make a positive impact in the lives of others. However, it is important for survivors to prioritize self-care and support while supporting others.

Childhood trauma can have significant and long-lasting effects on a person's physical, emotional, and mental health. Traumatic experiences in childhood, such as abuse, neglect, or witnessing violence, can result in a range of negative outcomes, including anxiety, depression, post-traumatic stress disorder, substance abuse, and physical health problems.

The impact of childhood trauma can be especially profound because it occurs during a crucial period of development when the brain is still developing and shaping. Trauma can interfere with healthy brain development, which can lead to problems with emotion regulation, decision-making, and interpersonal relationships.

Fortunately, healing and recovery are possible with appropriate support and interventions. Therapy, support groups, and other forms of professional help can assist individuals in processing and managing their traumatic experiences. It is also essential to prioritize self-care, engage in healthy coping strategies, and establish healthy relationships to promote healing and resilience.

Overall, childhood trauma is a serious issue that requires attention, understanding, and support. It is important to recognize the impact of trauma and work to address it to help individuals lead healthy and fulfilling lives.

THE IMPORTANCE OF BREAKING THE SILENCE ON CHILDHOOD TRAUMA

Breaking the silence on childhood trauma is critically important for a number of reasons. Here are a few key ones:

- **It helps survivors heal:** For many survivors of childhood trauma, speaking out about what happened to them can be a crucial step towards healing. It allows them to confront the trauma they experienced, process their emotions and feelings, and begin to move forward in their lives.

- **It reduces stigma:** Unfortunately, many survivors of childhood trauma feel ashamed or embarrassed about what happened to them, and may worry that others will judge them or view them differently if they speak out. By breaking the silence and sharing their stories, survivors can help reduce the stigma and shame associated with childhood trauma, and encourage others to seek help and support.

- **It raises awareness:** When survivors speak out about their experiences, it can help raise awareness about the prevalence and impact of childhood trauma. This can help to educate the public, policymakers, and healthcare providers about the importance of addressing childhood trauma, and the need for effective prevention and treatment strategies.

- **It can help prevent future trauma:** By speaking out about their experiences and advocating for change, survivors of childhood trauma can help prevent future generations from experiencing similar trauma. This can include advocating for policies and programs that support children's mental health and wellbeing, as well as raising awareness about the signs and symptoms of childhood trauma so that others can recognize and respond to it effectively.

- **It can help survivors feel less alone:** Childhood trauma can be an isolating experience, and survivors may feel like they are the only ones who have gone through it. By speaking out, survivors can connect with others who have had similar experiences and find a sense of community and support.

- **It can encourage others to speak out:** When survivors speak out about their experiences, it can inspire others to do the same. This can help create a ripple effect of healing and empowerment, as more and more people break the silence and share their stories.

- **It can hold perpetrators accountable:** When survivors speak out about the abuse they experienced, it can help hold perpetrators accountable for their actions. This can include pursuing legal action, but it can also mean speaking out publicly and raising awareness about the harm caused by childhood trauma.

- **It can promote systemic change:** When survivors speak out about their experiences, it can draw attention to the systemic issues that contribute to childhood trauma, such as poverty, inequality, and social injustice. This can help spur policy changes and reforms that address these underlying issues and create a more just and equitable society.

In summary, breaking the silence on childhood trauma is important for many reasons. It can help survivors heal, reduce stigma, raise awareness, prevent future trauma, promote community, inspire others, hold perpetrators accountable, and promote systemic change.

Overall, breaking the silence on childhood trauma is a powerful way to promote healing, reduce stigma, raise awareness, and prevent future trauma. It is an important step towards creating a world where all children can grow up safe, healthy, and happy.

Support for Childhood Trauma

Resources and support for overcoming childhood trauma:

Childhood trauma can have a significant impact on a person's mental health and well-being. However, there are resources and support available to help individuals overcome their trauma and move forward with their lives. Here are some resources and support options that may be helpful:

- **Therapy:** A therapist can help individuals work through their childhood trauma in a safe and supportive environment. There are different types of therapy that may be effective, including cognitive behavioral therapy, trauma-focused therapy, and eye movement desensitization and reprocessing (EMDR).
- **Support groups:** Joining a support group can be helpful for individuals who have experienced childhood trauma. Being around others who have had similar

experiences can help individuals feel less alone and provide a sense of community and support.

- **Mindfulness practices:** Mindfulness practices, such as meditation and yoga, can help individuals manage their emotions and reduce stress and anxiety.

- **Hotlines and crisis support:** There are hotlines and crisis support services available for individuals who need immediate help. The National Child Traumatic Stress Network (NCTSN) has a list of resources for individuals who have experienced childhood trauma.

- **Online resources:** There are numerous online resources available for individuals who have experienced childhood trauma, including blogs, podcasts, and videos. The NCTSN and the National Institute of Mental Health (NIMH) both have extensive online resources for individuals seeking information and support.

- **Art therapy:** Art therapy is a type of therapy that uses creative expression, such as drawing, painting, or sculpting, to help individuals work through their emotions and heal from trauma.

- **EMDR therapy:** EMDR therapy is a type of therapy that uses eye movements or other forms of bilateral stimulation to help individuals process traumatic memories and reduce the intensity of their emotional reactions.

- **Medication:** In some cases, medication may be helpful for individuals who have experienced childhood trauma and are struggling with symptoms such as depression, anxiety, or post-traumatic stress disorder (PTSD).

- **Trauma-informed care:** Trauma-informed care is an approach to healthcare that recognizes the impact of trauma on individuals and seeks to create a safe and supportive environment for healing. This can be helpful for individuals seeking medical or mental health care.

- **Advocacy organizations:** There are many advocacy organizations that provide resources and support for individuals who have experienced childhood trauma, such as the National Association of Adult Survivors of Child Abuse (NAASCA) and the Child Mind Institute.

- **Self-help books:** There are many self-help books available that can provide information and guidance for individuals who have experienced childhood trauma. **Some popular titles include "The Body Keeps the Score" by Bessel van der Kolk and "Complex PTSD: From Surviving to Thriving" by Pete Walker.**

Remember that seeking help is a sign of strength, and there is no shame in asking for support when dealing with childhood trauma. It's important to find the resources and support that work best for you, and to be patient and kind to yourself as you work through your healing journey.

It's important to note that everyone's healing journey is different, and there is no one-size-fits-all solution for overcoming childhood trauma. It may take time, patience, and a combination of different resources and support to find what works best for each individual.

CONCLUSION

Childhood trauma can have a lasting impact on individuals, influencing their emotions, behavior, and even their physical health. Trauma can be caused by various events, including abuse, neglect, or witnessing violence. The effects of childhood trauma can persist into adulthood, leading to a range of mental health issues, including anxiety, depression, and post-traumatic stress disorder (PTSD).

The trauma trap refers to the tendency for individuals to become stuck in patterns of negative thinking and behavior that are driven by their childhood trauma. This trap can be challenging to break free from, but it is possible. Through therapy, self-reflection, and a commitment to change, individuals can unlock the trauma trap and move forward in their lives.

The first step in breaking free from the trauma trap is acknowledging that the trauma exists and recognizing how it has impacted your life. This can be a difficult process, as many individuals may have buried their trauma deep within themselves in an effort to cope. However, facing the trauma head-on is necessary to move forward.

Therapy can be a useful tool in unlocking the trauma trap. A trained therapist can help individuals understand how their trauma has influenced their behavior, thoughts, and emotions. They can also provide support as individuals work through the trauma and learn healthy coping mechanisms.

Self-reflection is also crucial in breaking free from the trauma trap. This involves taking a close look at your thoughts, emotions, and behaviors and identifying those that may be influenced by the trauma. Once these patterns are recognized, individuals can work to change them and develop healthier coping mechanisms.

One common trap that individuals who have experienced childhood trauma fall into is the belief that they are not worthy of love or care. This belief can lead to self-destructive behavior, such as substance abuse, self-harm, or engaging in unhealthy relationships. However, recognizing that this belief is a result of the trauma and not a reflection of their true worth can help individuals begin to break free from this pattern.

It is also essential to surround oneself with supportive people who can provide encouragement and validation as individuals work to break free from the trauma trap. This can include friends, family members, or support groups for individuals who have experienced trauma.

In addition to therapy and self-reflection, engaging in self-care can also help individuals break free from the trauma trap. This can involve activities that promote physical and emotional well-being, such as exercise, meditation, or spending time in nature.

Breaking free from the trauma trap is not an easy process, and it can take time and effort. However, it is possible, and the benefits of doing so are significant. By unlocking the trauma trap, individuals can free themselves from patterns of negative thinking and behavior that have been holding them back and move forward in their lives with a greater sense of self-worth and resilience.

In conclusion, childhood trauma can have a lasting impact on individuals, but it is possible to break free from the trauma trap. Acknowledging the trauma, seeking therapy, engaging in self-reflection, surrounding oneself with supportive people, and engaging in self-care can all help individuals break free from the chains of childhood trauma. By doing so, individuals

can live more fulfilling lives and experience a greater sense of
well-being.

REFERENCES

National Child Traumatic Stress Network. (2017). Childhood trauma and its effects: Implications for police. https://www.nctsn.org/sites/default/files/resources//childhood_trauma_and_its_effects_implications_for_police.pdf

McLaughlin, K. A., Sheridan, M. A., & Lambert, H. K. (2014). Childhood adversity and neural development: A systematic review. Annual Review of Developmental Psychology, 10(1), 277-301.

Felitti, V. J., Anda, R. F., Nordenberg, D., Williamson, D. F., Spitz, A. M., Edwards, V., ... & Marks, J. S. (1998). Relationship of childhood abuse and household dysfunction to many of the leading causes of death in adults: The Adverse Childhood Experiences (ACE) Study. American Journal of Preventive Medicine, 14(4), 245-258.

Anda, R. F., Felitti, V. J., Bremner, J. D., Walker, J. D., Whitfield, C., Perry, B. D., ... & Giles, W. H. (2006). The enduring effects of abuse and related adverse experiences in childhood: A convergence of evidence from neurobiology and epidemiology. European Archives of Psychiatry and Clinical Neuroscience, 256(3), 174-186.

Widom, C. S., Czaja, S. J., & Dutton, M. A. (2008). Childhood victimization and lifetime revictimization. Child Abuse & Neglect, 32(8), 785-796.

McLaughlin, K. A., Green, J. G., Gruber, M. J., Sampson, N. A., Zaslavsky, A. M., & Kessler, R. C. (2012). Childhood adversities and adult psychiatric disorders in the National Comorbidity Survey Replication I: Associations with first onset of DSM-IV disorders. Archives of General Psychiatry, 69(11), 113-123.

National Child Traumatic Stress Network. (2017). The essential elements of trauma-informed care. https://www.nctsn.org/sites/default/files/resources//essential_elements_of_trauma_informed_care.pdf

Substance Abuse and Mental Health Services Administration. (2014). Trauma-informed approach and trauma-specific interventions. Treatment Improvement Protocol (TIP) Series, No. 57. https://store.samhsa.gov/sites/default/files/d7/priv/sma14-4816.pdf

American Psychological Association. (2013). Guidelines for psychological practice with lesbian, gay, and bisexual clients.

American Psychologist, 68(9), 429-441. https://doi.org/10.1037/a0033999

Resick, P. A., & Schnicke, M. K. (1992). Cognitive processing therapy for sexual assault victims. Journal of Consulting and Clinical Psychology, 60(5), 748-756. https://doi.org/10.1037/0022-006X.60.5.748

Felitti, V. J., Anda, R. F., Nordenberg, D., Williamson, D. F., Spitz, A. M., Edwards, V., ... & Marks, J. S. (1998). Relationship of childhood abuse and household dysfunction to many of the leading causes of death in adults: The Adverse Childhood Experiences (ACE) Study. American Journal of Preventive Medicine, 14(4), 245-258. https://doi.org/10.1016/s0749-3797(98)00017-8

Centers for Disease Control and Prevention. (2022). Adverse Childhood Experiences (ACEs). https://www.cdc.gov/violenceprevention/aces/index.html

Anda, R. F., Felitti, V. J., Bremner, J. D., Walker, J. D., Whitfield, C., Perry, B. D., ... & Giles, W. H. (2006). The enduring effects of abuse and related adverse experiences in childhood. European Archives of Psychiatry and Clinical

Neuroscience, 256(3), 174-186. https://doi.org/10.1007/s00406-005-0624-4

Brown, D. W., Anda, R. F., Tiemeier, H., Felitti, V. J., Edwards, V. J., Croft, J. B., & Giles, W. H. (2009). Adverse childhood experiences and the risk of premature mortality. American Journal of Preventive Medicine, 37(5), 389-396. https://doi.org/10.1016/j.amepre.2009.06.021

Hughes, K., Bellis, M. A., Hardcastle, K. A., Sethi, D., Butchart, A., Mikton, C., ... & Dunne, M. P. (2017). The effect of multiple adverse childhood experiences on health: a systematic review and meta-analysis. The Lancet Public Health, 2(8), e356-e366. https://doi.org/10.1016/S2468-2667(17)30118-4

Cohen, J. A., Deblinger, E., Mannarino, A. P., & Steer, R. A. (2004). A multisite, randomized controlled trial for children with sexual abuse-related PTSD symptoms. Journal of the American Academy of Child & Adolescent Psychiatry, 43(4), 393-402. doi: 10.1097/00004583-200404000-00004

Deblinger, E., Mannarino, A. P., Cohen, J. A., Runyon, M. K., & Steer, R. A. (2011). Trauma-focused cognitive behavioral therapy for children: Impact of the trauma narrative and treatment length. Depression and Anxiety, 28(1), 67-75. doi: 10.1002/da.20743

Lester, K. J., Roberts, S., Keers, R., Coleman, J. R. I., Breen, G., Wong, C. C. Y., . . . Eley, T. C. (2016). Non-replication of the association between 5HTTLPR and response to psychological therapy for child anxiety disorders. British Journal of Psychiatry, 208(2), 182-188. doi: 10.1192/bjp.bp.114.161836

McLean, C. P., Morris, S. H., Conklin, P., Jayawickreme, N., & Foa, E. B. (2014). Trauma characteristics and posttraumatic stress disorder among adolescent survivors of childhood sexual abuse. Journal of Family Violence, 29(7), 701-710. doi: 10.1007/s10896-014-9639-9

Murray, L. K., Skavenski, S., Bass, J., Wilcox, H. C., Bolton, P., Imasiku, M., . . . Cohen, J. A. (2014). Implementing evidence-based mental health care in low-resource settings: A focus on safety planning procedures. Journal of Cognitive Psychotherapy, 28(2), 148-163. doi: 10.1891/0889-8391.28.2.148

Shapiro, F. (2014). The role of eye movement desensitization and reprocessing (EMDR) therapy in medicine: addressing the psychological and physical symptoms stemming from adverse life experiences. The Permanente Journal, 18(1), 71–77. https://doi.org/10.7812/TPP/13-098

de Roos, C., Veenstra, A. C., de Jongh, A., den Hollander-Gijsman, M., van der Wee, N. J., & Zitman, F. G. (2011). Treatment of chronic phantom limb pain using a trauma-focused psychological approach. Pain Research and Treatment, 2011, 1–7. https://doi.org/10.1155/2011/754864

Greenwald, R. (2018). Eye movement desensitization and reprocessing (EMDR) therapy in the treatment of traumatized individuals. Journal of Psychology and Clinical Psychiatry, 8(3), 1–4. https://doi.org/10.15406/jpcpy.2018.08.00323

Harned, M. S. (2018). Dialectical behavior therapy for the treatment of trauma-related disorders. In J. L. Tull, M. J. Roemer, & K. A. Walsh (Eds.), Handbook of Dialectical Behavior Therapy: Theory, Research, and Evaluation (pp. 223-243). Guilford Press.

Cohen, J. N., & Mannarino, A. P. (2018). Trauma-focused cognitive-behavioral therapy and dialectical behavior therapy. Child and Adolescent Psychiatric Clinics of North America, 27(2), 165-176.

Kliem, S., Kroger, C., & Kosfelder, J. (2010). Dialectical behavior therapy for posttraumatic stress disorder related to childhood sexual abuse: A pilot study of an intensive residential treatment program. Journal of Traumatic Stress, 23(1), 137-146.

Cohen, J. A., Deblinger, E., Mannarino, A. P., & Steer, R. A. (2004). A multisite, randomized controlled trial for children with sexual abuse-related PTSD symptoms. Journal of the American Academy of Child and Adolescent Psychiatry, 43(4), 393-402.

This randomized controlled trial evaluated the effectiveness of TF-CBT for children who had experienced sexual abuse-related PTSD symptoms. The study found that TF-CBT was significantly more effective than a waitlist control group in reducing PTSD symptoms, depression, and anxiety.

Shedler, J. (2010). The efficacy of psychodynamic psychotherapy. American Psychologist, 65(2), 98–109. https://doi.org/10.1037/a0018378

Fonagy, P., Target, M., & Allison, E. (2015). The implications of attachment theory and research for understanding borderline personality disorder. Development and

Psychopathology, 27(4pt1), 1091–1104. https://doi.org/10.1017/S095457941500068X

Perry, J. C. (2011). Psychodynamic therapy for personality pathology: A systematic review of empirical evidence. Harvard Review of Psychiatry, 19(5), 245–255. https://doi.org/10.3109/10673229.2011.614601

Emerson, D., Sharma, R., Chaudhry, S., & Turner, J. (2009). Trauma-sensitive yoga: Principles, practice, and research. International Journal of Yoga Therapy, 19(1), 123-128.

van der Kolk, B. A., Stone, L., West, J., Rhodes, A., Emerson, D., Suvak, M., ... & Spinazzola, J. (2014). Yoga as an adjunctive treatment for posttraumatic stress disorder: A randomized controlled trial. Journal of Clinical Psychiatry, 75(6), e559-e565.

Goldin, P. R., & Gross, J. J. (2010). Effects of mindfulness-based stress reduction (MBSR) on emotion regulation in social anxiety disorder. Emotion, 10(1), 83–91.

Kim, M., Lee, Y., Kim, E., & Kim, Y. (2018). The effects of trauma-focused yoga on posttraumatic stress disorder symptoms and distress tolerance. Journal of Psychiatric and Mental Health Nursing, 25(6), 357-366.

Telles, S., Singh, N., Joshi, M., & Balkrishna, A. (2010). Post-traumatic stress symptoms and heart rate variability in Bihar flood survivors following yoga: A randomized controlled study. BMC Psychiatry, 10(1), 18.